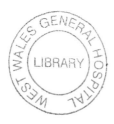

D1575105

# Cutting to the Core

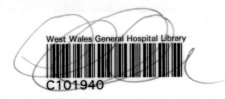

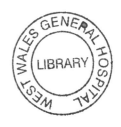

# Cutting to the Core

## Exploring the Ethics of Contested Surgeries

Edited by
David Benatar

ROWMAN & LITTLEFIELD PUBLISHERS, INC.
*Lanham • Boulder • New York • Toronto • Oxford*

ROWMAN & LITTLEFIELD PUBLISHERS, INC.

Published in the United States of America
by Rowman & Littlefield Publishers, Inc.
A wholly owned subsidiary of The Rowman & Littlefield Publishing Group, Inc.
4501 Forbes Boulevard, Suite 200, Lanham, Maryland 20706
www.rowmanlittlefield.com

PO Box 317
Oxford
OX2 9RU, UK

British Library Cataloguing in Publication Information Available

**Library of Congress Cataloging-in-Publication Data**

Cutting to the core : exploring the ethics of contested surgeries / edited by David
Benatar.
    p. cm.
Includes bibliographical references and index.
ISBN-13: 978-0-7425-5000-1 (cloth : alk. paper)
ISBN-10: 0-7425-5000-1 (cloth : alk. paper)
ISBN-13: 978-0-7425-5001-8 (pbk. : alk. paper)
ISBN-10: 0-7425-5001-X (pbk. : alk. paper)
1. Surgery—Moral and ethical aspects. 2. Medical ethics. I. Benatar, David.
RD27.7.C87 2006
174'.9617—dc22                                                                    2005028842

Printed in the United States of America

♾ ™ The paper used in this publication meets the minimum requirements of
American National Standard for Information Sciences—Permanence of Paper for
Printed Library Materials, ANSI/NISO Z39.48-1992.

To my father, Solomon,
and my brother, Michael.

One a pulmonologist; the other a neurologist.
Neither a surgeon.

# Contents

# Preface

By its own lights, the adage *primum non nocere* ("first, do no harm") is the first principle of medical practice. For this principle to have any application to surgery, the relevant sense of "harm" must be understood to be "all things considered." This is because surgery inevitably involves harm in another, more basic sense—damage to the tissue that is cut. Surgeons take the knife (and other instruments of cutting) to living flesh and bone. In doing so, they damage that flesh and bone. If they are to conform to a requirement to do no harm, then the damaged tissue must not constitute a harm from some more general perspective that considers not only the effect on the tissue but also on the patient as a whole. An incision to excise a tumor, for example, damages the incised tissue but, one hopes, saves the patient.

Where a surgical intervention is plausibly aimed at yielding a net benefit, it is usually uncontested. In cases of competent patients, the only rider is that the patient must consent, because even beneficial surgery performed without the consent of a competent patient is wrong. Surgeries become contested—defended by some and opposed by others—when it is doubtful whether a net benefit is produced. In cases of competent patients, it is asked whether surgeons may respect a patient's informed consent to a surgical intervention that is unlikely to produce a net benefit and may even be a harm. The concern arises *a fortiori* in cases of incompetent patients. Given that they cannot consent, their wishes cannot even enter into the equation and thus cannot be thought to override their interests in avoiding a surgical intervention that is not beneficial and may be harmful.

This book examines a number of contested surgeries. These include infant male circumcision and cutting the genitals of female children, the separation of conjoined twins, surgical sex assignment of intersex children and the surgical sex reassignment of transsexuals, limb and face transplantation, cosmetic surgery, and placebo surgery.

Although the authors writing for this volume have not sought to provide new scientific data about the benefits or harms of these surgeries, many of them have drawn on the available data and incorporated this information into their ethical discussions of the contested surgeries.

The intended readership of this book includes surgeons, who are invited to reflect on their practices (and on practices they may be avoiding), students and scholars of bioethics, and laypeople of various kinds. The latter may include those who are affected in some way—parents who are considering circumcising their child, parents of conjoined twins or intersex children, amputees considering a limb transplant, or people contemplating a face transplant or cosmetic surgery. But the lay readers may also include interested members of the general public who, although not personally affected, want to learn more about the ethics of any one of these procedures. Accordingly, although the authors are mostly philosophers (but also include a few lawyers, a social scientist, and a doctor or two), the chapters do not presuppose any philosophical or other training. They are intended to be generally accessible.

In the introduction that follows this preface, I introduce the reader to the book's theme and discuss the book's scope and content. I then provide an overview of the surgeries that will be discussed and present some of the relevant issues. Finally, I highlight some recurring ethical themes.

Most of the chapters in this volume have been written especially for this collection. I am grateful to the authors for their contributions.

As always, my thanks go to my parents and brothers. This book is dedicated to the two doctors among them. I have learned much about medicine from them and they have come to share my interest in philosophy and ethics. We have collaborated in teaching and writing about bioethics. It has been a pleasure to work with them at the intersection of our professional interests.

# Introduction: The Ethics of Contested Surgeries

## David Benatar

There is an important but often fine line between surgery and assault. That line is marked, at least in the case of patients competent to make decisions for themselves, by informed and voluntary consent. Where such consent is present, assault is absent. In the absence of this consent, surgery becomes assault (even if it benefits the patient). However, the ethics of surgery is not simply about the avoidance of assault. This is true not only in the case of those who lack the competence to consent to or to refuse surgery—cases in which decisions must be made in accordance with the best interests of the patient. Even where patients are competent to give informed consent, the best-interests standards may not be entirely voided. Surgeons, it seems to some people, should avoid inflicting (at least serious) harm, even if the patient consents to the harm.

Particular surgeries become morally contested where there is doubt about how their benefits weigh up against their harms, some people believing that the latter are greater than the former, while others disagreeing. The contestation is heightened when candidates for the surgery are incompetent to decide whether it should be performed on them.

Given that much of the controversy rests on the question of whether some surgical procedure does more harm or more good, establishing the facts is a substantial part of resolving the moral question. It is notoriously difficult, however, to answer these empirical questions. There are many reasons for this. The science is often difficult and the evidence equivocal. Compounding these problems is the ideological agenda or other bias that many people bring to either the empirical investigation or the interpretation of the results. Far too few people approach these questions agnostically and let themselves be led wherever the evidence takes them.

The ethics of contested surgeries is not merely about determining harms and benefits, however. Partly because of the aforementioned bias, but also partly because of the pervasiveness of sloppy thinking, the moral waters are muddied by conceptual and other confusion. These waters need to be cleared. Moreover, there are many moral questions that need to be confronted. For instance, how should we react to equivocal evidence about the harms and benefits? Just how autonomous must consent be? What are the moral limits, if any, of even fully autonomous consent? To what extent should cultural and societal norms be taken as a given and to what extent should they be challenged? Should an incompetent's best interests be determined within a cultural context or independent of it?

The chapters in this volume do not purport to offer any new empirical evidence about the harms and benefits of the surgical procedures that are discussed. However, the chapters are empirically informed. Their authors have attempted to seek out and report the best evidence. This is woven into conceptual and moral arguments that seek to shed light on the ethics of contested surgeries. Most, but not all, of these surgeries cut to the core. Some, such as male circumcision and some forms of placebo surgery, involve more superficial incisions. However, the "cutting to the core" that entitles this volume refers not to the surgeries themselves but rather to the kind of analysis and argument necessary to assess their ethical status.

This enterprise requires the questioning of common assumptions. This is not to say that common assumptions are always wrong, although it is also highly unlikely that they are always correct. The assumptions need to be questioned and tested. Some may remain standing, while others may fall.

## THE SCOPE AND CONTENT OF THIS BOOK

There are more contested surgeries than can be examined in a book of reasonable length. Accordingly, choices about what to include and what to exclude have had to be made. I have chosen a range of procedures. Most, despite being contested, are either relatively common or widely accepted. Others are either quite uncommon or widely viewed with suspicion, if not actively opposed. In other words, questions will be raised as to whether certain common or accepted surgeries should continue to be performed, and whether some surgeries that are uncommon or widely opposed should become accepted, or at least tolerated.

A number of contested surgeries have been excluded because the moral issues are not essentially about the surgery itself. Thus there is no discussion of abortion procedures, such as the highly contested "partial birth" abortion (known medically, if also euphemistically, as intact dilation and extraction). Although this involves a surgical procedure—puncturing and collapsing the head of the fetus—the core moral issues pertain to the moral status of the fetus. Similarly excluded is any discussion of experimental surgery performed on animals. The moral issues here pertain to experimentation on animals and not specifically to *surgical* experimentation.

Other surgeries not included are limb lengthening for children with achondroplasia and facial surgery to fashion more normal features in children with Down's syndrome (Trisomy-21). Although these surgeries each raise a unique combination of issues, some of these same issues also arise in connection with surgeries that *are* covered in the book. For instance, they raise questions about normality and the extent to which surgery should be employed in its pursuit. This question is discussed in the chapters on the separation of conjoined twins and in the chapter on the surgical treatment of intersex children.

Another issue raised by facial surgery on Trisomy-21 children is that of cosmetic surgery. A more normal-looking face does not undo mental retardation or extend life span. Although there are chapters on cosmetic surgery in this book, those discussions are of either limited or contested application to the cosmetic surgery on Trisomy-21 children. This is because the cosmetic surgeries discussed in this book are not cosmetic normalization surgery but rather primarily "enhancements" above normality. By way of example, breast reconstruction following mastectomy would be an instance of normalization, whereas augmentation of healthy breasts that are perceived to be "too small" is an "enhancement." The distinction between normalization and enhancement is controversial. Some deny that a sharp line can be drawn between them. Others suggest that even if they can be distinguished, the distinction is not of moral significance.

Another, and unusual, kind of cosmetic surgery not discussed in this book is hymen reconstruction.[1] This relatively rare form of surgery is intended to create the impression of virginity. This could be performed on a girl or woman who is no longer a virgin, as a result of having had sexual intercourse (consensual or otherwise), but it could also be performed on a virgin whose hymen was ruptured accidentally. Some issues raised by this surgery, such as deception, are not raised by any of the surgeries that are discussed.[2] However, other issues relevant to hymen restoration also arise in other surgeries. For example, to what extent should we use surgery to pander to questionable societal values—whether it be undue emphasis on the *signs* of virginity or undue emphasis on breast size?

Still more outlandish than hymen reconstruction is the amputation of healthy limbs. This topic too is not examined in this book. Some readers may think that such surgery is *obviously* wrong and thus not a candidate for a *contested* surgery. However, that judgment is too hasty. Those who defend such surgery can argue that it is the most effective treatment for people who have what has been known (most commonly) as either apotemnophilia[3] or body integrity identity disorder.[4] Those who have this condition are colloquially known as "wannabes"[5]—what they want to be is an amputee. This is not the result of a delusion,[6] and the desire may not be eliminable without actually fulfilling it. Some wannabes have performed amputations on themselves or inflicted injuries on themselves that have resulted in amputation. However, others have persuaded surgeons to amputate healthy limbs.[7] The most well-known recent case is that of Dr. Robert Smith, a Scottish surgeon, who conducted amputations on two wannabes and was poised to operate on a third when he was stopped.[8] Some of the issues raised by body integrity identity disorder[9] parallel those in gender identity disorder and are thus discussed in the chapter on sex reassignment that appears in this book.

Other forms of contested surgery not covered in this book are those procedures, such as gastric bypass, that treat obesity by inhibiting appetite. Such procedures are surgical ways of making dieting and weight loss easier. Some of the opposition to these surgeries is a Spartan intolerance of "weakness" and of "easy ways out." The more compelling concerns, however, have to do with the safety and morbidity of these practices and the question of whether these are worth the benefits. Although the empirical questions of harms and benefits in these particular surgeries are not discussed in this book, the more conceptual and normative issues also arise in cosmetic surgery, which is discussed.

Each section of this book is devoted to a different contested surgery or to two related surgeries: Part 1 discusses male circumcision and female genital cutting. In part 2, attention is given to sex assignment of intersex children and sex reassignment of those who believe that they occupy a body of the wrong sex. Part 3 is devoted to the separation of conjoined twins. In part 4, limb and face transplantations are examined. Cosmetic surgery is the subject of part 5. Finally, part 6 considers placebo surgery.

In those sections in which more than one chapter is devoted to a single surgery, the aim has *not* been to secure one "for" and one "against" the contested surgery. That format, although it has its merits, can produce stilted results and create undue polarization. Sometimes the difference between the most plausible positions on some question is less marked and more nuanced. In soliciting chapters, I *have* sought to have differing views or approaches represented, but in some cases, although the approaches differ, the conclusions do not.

Each section of this book is devoted to a different kind of contested surgery (or set of surgeries), though there are obviously intersections between some of them. Thus, for example, sex assignment surgery involves genital cutting. Separating conjoined twins may sometimes entail reassigning the sex of one of the twins.

## MALE CIRCUMCISION AND FEMALE GENITAL CUTTING

Male circumcision, arguably the mildest of surgeries discussed in this book,[10] is nearly unknown in some countries and widely practiced in others.

In most places where it is practiced, it is performed for either cultural or religious reasons, but there are some places where the high incidence is attributable to other factors. In the United States, for example, it was once taken to be medically desirable. Although the medical community is now more equivocal about its benefits, the practice has become sufficiently entrenched that many people circumcise their sons because it strikes them as the normal thing to do—just as normal as not circumcising is in societies to which the practice is foreign.

Where circumcision is not ignored, it is most commonly thought to be morally acceptable. It is regarded as a minor surgical procedure that, even if it does not advance the interests of the child on whom it is performed, does not run counter to his interests either. However, there is a small but vocal group of opponents who view circumcision as mutilation and, when it is performed on minors, a form of child abuse.[11] They deny that it holds any benefits and claim that it inflicts significant harm. At the opposite end of the spectrum are those who hold that circumcision is strongly indicated medically—that it bestows significant benefits and, although carrying a very small risk of harm, is almost always harmless.

In our chapter, Michael Benatar and I argue that neither of these positions is convincing. While the intermediate view is not the correct one in *every* controversy, our assessment of the medical evidence and moral arguments suggests that in the case of neonatal male circumcision an intermediate view is the right one. We argue that although routine male circumcision is not medically indicated, it is also not contraindicated. This book does not include a contribution from any of the extreme opponents or proponents of circumcision. Because the truth seems to lie in the intermediate ground, it made sense to include a chapter opposed to ours not from the extremes, but rather from elsewhere in the center. In her chapter, Leslie Cannold defends a moderate opposition to circumcision.

I purposely avoided entitling part 1 "Circumcision" or "Male and Female Circumcision," because although circumcision is an apt description of the procedure performed on males, the genital cutting most commonly performed on females is a much more radical procedure. Its opponents have preferred to dub it "female genital mutilation." Because that term is tendentious and normatively laden, however, I prefer to avoid it, too. We may decide that it is wrong, but it is best not to presuppose that outcome in naming the very practice we are still evaluating. Thus I prefer the neutral term, "female genital cutting," which is neither condemnatory nor euphemistic. Dena Davis, who wrote on this topic for this volume, uses the term "genital alteration," which is a similarly neutral term.

Female genital cutting is a much more variable procedure than removal of the foreskin in male circumcision. It may entail as little as nicking the clitoral prepuce or as much as excising the clitoris and labia minora and majora and then infibulating the girl or woman by stitching together the remaining tissue, allowing a small hole for the passage of urine and menstrual blood. In practice, the procedure is rarely less severe than the partial or complete excision of the clitoris, and very often much more severe. The degree of severity is commonly classified into one of four types. Unfortunately, however, the taxonomies differ significantly,[12] making them rather less helpful than they otherwise would be.

Although female genital cutting is accepted by many (but not all) in those societies in which it is practiced, it is generally condemned elsewhere. Critics of the practice say that in addition to the short-term sequelae, such as excruciating pain, hemorrhaging, and wound infection, there are longer-term sequelae, including urinary tract infections, dysmenorrhea, and diminished sexual pleasure if not painful sexual intercourse. Such lists convince many people, but there are some scholars who have questioned how representative these possible consequences are of all female genital cutting.[13] They are certainly absent in the mildest versions—in which the clitoris is merely nicked—yet shrill and effective opposition has prevented even this form of female genital cutting being practiced in a number of Western societies.[14] Although there are much stronger grounds for condemning the more severe forms of female genital cutting, it is hard to see how the mildest forms could be condemned, particularly if male circumcision, a more severe procedure, is accepted.

## SEX ASSIGNMENT AND REASSIGNMENT

Many people assume that there are only two sexes—female and male. Although it is true that the overwhelming majority of people do fall into one of these two categories, there are a significant number of people who do not fit neatly into either category. These people have been known by a variety of names, including "hermaphrodite" and the now more common and preferred "intersex" person.[15]

Intersex is a not a single condition but can be the consequence of a number of genetic and endocrine abnormalities.[16] For example, girls with classic congenital adrenal hyperplasia (CAH) typically manifest some degree of virilization of the external genitalia, even though their internal female sexual organs (uterus, fallopian tubes, and ovaries) are normal.[17] Genetic males with androgen insensitivity syndrome (AIS) have female external genitalia, develop breasts, and are like women in having little body hair. However, they have (undescended) testes rather than ovaries, do not menstruate, and cannot bear children. Genetic males with 5-alpha-reductase deficiency appear female at birth but transform to male appearance at puberty. Other conditions also causing some degree of sexual ambiguity include Klinefelter's syndrome and Turner's syndrome.

As might be suspected from the above range of conditions, intersex sometimes becomes apparent only at puberty. However, there certainly are cases of intersex that are apparent at birth. These infants are often surgically assigned, within the first year or two of life, to either male or female sex. The usual justification for this is to spare the intersex child a sense of abnormality, to avoid it becoming an object of morbid curiosity, thereby causing it shame, and to prevent the discomfort attendant upon being neither male nor female.

Although the intention of surgical assignment may be to serve the child's best interest, it is far from clear that it always has this effect. There is now a growing and powerful challenge to the practice. In the first place, it has been noted that gender—psychological sex—is not quite as plastic as was once thought. A child reared in one sex will not necessarily adopt the corresponding gender identity.[18] Other factors, most notably hormonal ones, play a crucial role. Second, intersex people have been critical of sex-assignment surgery that was performed on them as infants. For many of them, this surgery has limited their capacity for sexual pleasure, which although unimportant to an infant or child, is important to the adult that child becomes. Moreover, they question the necessity of assigning intersex children to either male or female sex. Even if it is true that intersex children and adults occupy some twilight zone between the two (common) sexes, the appropriate response to this, they say, is not surgical and hormonal intervention, but rather societal change. In other words, the bodies of intersex children should not be altered to fit the societal assumption that the correct taxonomy of sex is binary. Instead, the taxonomy of sex should be molded to fit the natural reality—that some people are neither male nor female.

When one considers just how expansive and forceful the grip of the current classification is, this is no small task. To undo entirely the dichotomous thinking about sex would require either removing questions about a person's sex on government and other forms, or adding a third option (if that were not deemed a violation of privacy).[19] It would require either the elimination of gendered pronouns or the addition of another one. It would require the elimination of single-sex public toilets, changing rooms, and showers in favor of unisex ones.[20] It would require blurring the boundaries between heterosexuality and homosexuality. (If it is not clear whether somebody is male or female, then it is unclear whether that person's attraction to a male or female is heterosexual or homosexual.) That it would require all this plus much more does not undermine the value of aspiring to make society more accommodating of and sensitive to intersex people. Even if full accommodation cannot be attained, there is much that could be done.

In their contribution to this volume, Merle Spriggs and Julian Savulescu take up the question of whether intersex children should ever be assigned surgically to the male or female sex. They do not rule out the possibility that under some circumstances they should, but they correctly note that this depends heavily on whether early surgery benefits the child. They argue that we still have insufficient evidence to make a fully informed decision.

Whereas the bodies of intersex people are neither unambiguously male nor unambiguously female, the bodies of transsexuals quite clearly are either male or female. Transsexuals are those who believe themselves to be trapped in a body of the wrong sex. There is a discord between their bodily and psychological sex. This explains why some transsexuals seek surgical (and hormonal) sex reassignment. Heather Draper and Neil Evans discuss the question of whether requests for such reassignment should be fulfilled. They raise the question of whether transsexuals really are people of one sex trapped in the body of the opposite sex or are instead simply mistaken. The authors argue, however, that surgery may be warranted even if transsexuals are mistaken. Sex reassignment may be the most effective way of resolving their problem. But because this may not always be the case, the authors recommend caution in making such momentous decisions, and they suggest a number of precautions and safeguards.

## SEPARATING CONJOINED TWINS

There is a close parallel between sex assignment of intersex children and the separation of conjoined twins.[21] Just as the quest for normality drives many parents and surgeons to want their children to be unambiguously of one or other sex, so surgeons and parents are similarly driven to separate conjoined twins. The aim of separation is to give the children (or the surviving child) normal lives as separate people.

In the same way that the assumptions about the value of being normally sexed can be questioned, so we can question the assumption that being separate is so important. It is difficult for most people to question these assumptions. This is because people are so heavily influenced by the norm. Accordingly, it may help to imagine a world in which most people were conjoined, but a few were not. If the inhabitants of such a world were as driven by the impulse to normality that characterize the inhabitants of our world, they would seek not a surgical separation of the conjoined, but rather a surgical fusing of the separate. Just as we might pity conjoined twins their lack of independence and privacy, so they might pity the unconjoined's lack of the kind of companionship that they enjoy all the time.

This may sound implausible to proponents of separation. They might note that conjoined twins not only lack independence and privacy, but, depending on where they are joined, may also suffer from impeded mobility. However, whatever such disadvantages there may be, those conjoined twins who are not separated seem not to value separation sufficiently to overcome them. Most conjoined twins who are not separated as children are happy that they were not separated and want to remain joined.[22] This sometimes applies even when one of them dies and only separation can prevent the otherwise inevitable imminent death of the second.

Although these reflections should call into question the common assumption that living conjoined is an unmitigated harm and that separation should routinely be performed, they do not imply that separation is never permissible. I noted earlier that there is an interesting similarity between sex assignment of intersex children and the separation of conjoined twins. There appears, however, also to be an interesting difference between the two.[23] Although most conjoined twins who are not separated are pleased not to have been separated and prefer not to be separated, most of those conjoined twins who were separated are happy that they were so. This seems to stand in contrast to surgical disambiguation of sex, where many of those who were surgically assigned to one of the two sexes wish that they had not been subjected to the surgery. This difference makes the case for separation somewhat stronger than the case for surgical sex assignment. However, it is not sufficient to justify the surgery. For why should one privilege the preference of those who were separated over the preference of those who were not?

We also need to consider the costs of separation. These vary from case to case, but can be substantial. For example, in cases where conjoined twins have only two arms between them, separation will result in each twin having only one arm. If being conjoined is a disability, then so is having only one arm. In deciding whether to separate, one has to take such factors into account and weigh up the potential costs and benefits. This is true even if the twins would come to endorse whichever decision one made.

Not all instances of separation result in two separate people. Sometimes one or both of the twins die. This possibility has to be considered even when it is not foreseen as a likely outcome. There are also cases where the death of one of the twins is expected. In such cases, separation is harder to justify unless both twins would die if they were not separated. But even then separation remains controversial. Some people think that it is wrong to perform surgery that one knows will kill one twin, even though that is the only way to the save the other. Others, though they regret the death of the one twin, believe that the surgery is justified because in its absence *both* twins would die. Performing the surgery is pareto-optimal.

If twins are to be separated, one needs to ask *when* this should be done. There are those who think that we should wait, at least where this would not result in the death of the twins, until they reach majority and can make the decision for themselves. The problem with this is that the success of the surgery can vary depending on when it is performed. Although the timing that would maximize success varies, depending on the circumstances, the best time is often well before majority. Delaying separation is then to the detriment of the twins. In terms of the possible death of one or both of the twins, early separation is preferable. It is probably better to die during infancy than it is to die in early adulthood once one's interests in continued living have become quite robust.

In this volume, there are two chapters about the separation of conjoined twins. Both consider whether the state of being conjoined is a disability.

Richard Hull and Stephen Wilkinson also consider whether conjoined twins have a distinct moral-ontological status. David Wasserman considers how we might adjudicate conflicting interests of conjoined twins, both with regard to separation and if they remain conjoined. Neither chapter concludes that separation is always wrong. Nor do they conclude that separation surgery should be performed routinely. The authors of both chapters think that the pros and cons of separation have to be weighed, although it is not clear that they would evaluate them in the same way.

## LIMB AND FACE TRANSPLANTATION

It is a sad irony that while there are some people whose healthy limbs seem foreign to them and who wish them amputated, there are others who have lost limbs through disease or injury and would dearly love to have them restored. Limb transplantation is a recent development.[24] The first such transplant was performed in Lyon, France, in September 1998. The second took place in Louisville, Kentucky, in January the following year. Since then, many others have been performed. The procedure remains contested, however. At the time of writing, no face transplant has yet been performed, although the first seems relatively imminent. Face transplantation is even more contested than limb transplantation.

Transplantation of any kind involves considerable costs and risks to the recipient who has to be immunosuppressed in order to prevent rejection of the graft. Being immunosuppressed can feel unpleasant and puts one at risk not only for opportunistic infections but also for malignancies. These harms and risks are usually warranted because without the surgery the patient would die very soon. Heart and lung transplants, for example, save lives. The same is not true of limb and face transplants. Amputees' lives are not in danger. What limb transplantation offers them is the possibility of heightened, although not (yet) normal, functionality. Face transplantation offers those with horribly disfigured faces the opportunity for a more (but not entirely) normal-looking face. Because their disfigurement can have profound psychological and social costs, this benefit should not be underestimated. The common view is that the benefits are nonetheless not equivalent to saving a life. That view is disputable. Those amputees and facially disfigured people who ask for a limb or face transplant indicate a preference for assuming the harms and risks over continuing life without a limb or with a disfigured face. In doing so, they either think that the benefits *are* equivalent to saving a life, or they at least think that the benefits nevertheless warrant the risks. In making these judgments, it is possible for people to be mistaken, even relative to their own values. For example, the recipient of the first hand transplant eventually had the graft removed at his request (primarily because of "poor hand function and the side-effects of his immunosuppressive regime").[25]

This volume contains one chapter on limb transplantation and one on face transplants. In the former, Donna Dickenson and Guy Widdershoven argue that although limb transplantation raises deep moral dilemmas, it cannot be ruled out and may be justified in some circumstances. In her chapter, Françoise Baylis takes a stronger view against face transplantation. Although there are those who would want to oppose both limb and face transplantation, there is at least one difference between the two that makes the latter more troubling. Given that rejection remains a possibility even under a regime of immunosuppression, removing the graft may sometimes be necessary to prevent death. Although the process of transplanting and then amputating a limb does involve some loss of original tissues—first in the resection necessary for grafting and then in amputating above the graft line—the patient is still left with much of the original segment of limb. The problem with face transplantation is that it involves not simply addition of a graft, but also the prior removal of the recipient's face. Once that face, disfigured though it may be, has been removed, it is lost. If the graft is rejected, one cannot revert to the preoperative situation.

There is a further problem that once plagued limb transplantation and still confronts face transplantation. This is the obvious conflict of interest that a surgeon faces in pioneering a risky surgical innovation that is likely to bring some fame to the surgeon. History has been remarkably kind to pioneering surgeons who have caused great harm to their patients. If this is any indication of how people will react in the future, it is unlikely that the surgeons pioneering new and risky transplants will bear any costs of the failure. These costs will be borne exclusively by their patients (or, as Françoise Baylis would say, their research subjects). This calls, at least, for an elevated level of ethical scrutiny.

## COSMETIC SURGERY

Although face transplantation is a kind of cosmetic surgery, it is quite unlike the interventions that will be considered under the rubric of "cosmetic surgery" in this book. This is because face transplantation is aimed at ameliorating an extreme and unequivocal disfigurement. It is not contested because it aims at improving the patient's appearance, which is seen as a noble goal, but rather because its costs and risks are so extreme. Other cosmetic repairs of less serious deformities are largely uncontested primarily because the surgery is relatively low risk. But many other cosmetic surgical interventions with relatively low risks *do* face criticism. Rhinoplasty, face-lifts, breast enhancement or reduction, and penile enlargement, for example, are widely criticized, at least in part, for their aesthetic goals.

Setting aside such especially risky surgery as face transplantation, what differentiates those cosmetic procedures that are criticized from those that are not is a distinction between therapy and enhancement. The argument is that cosmetic surgery to fix a deformity or injury is acceptable, while cosmetic surgery to enhance a normal person is unacceptable. The distinction between therapy and enhancement has been challenged. It has been suggested, for example, that there is no sharp distinction between them—that it is often unclear whether some intervention is a treatment or an enhancement. For example, just how big or crooked does one's nose have to be before it is "deformed"? Just how big or protuberant must one's ears be to be candidates for "therapy" rather than "enhancement"? This is an important response to those critics of cosmetic surgery who oppose only cosmetic enhancement. Many of those who seek cosmetic surgery that some label "enhancement" may in fact be closer to "therapy."

Nevertheless, although the distinction may not be a sharp one, there does seem to be a moral difference between the extremes. The pursuit of mere enhancements may more plausibly be charged with being vain, obsessive, and a manifestation of shallow values. The better the trait before enhancement the more prone the pursuit of cosmetic surgery is to this criticism. Although vanity, obsessiveness, and shallowness may be vices, their motivating cosmetic surgery is not sufficient to show that cosmetic surgery is morally impermissible. There are many vain, obsessive, and shallow practices—such as concern about and repair of every little nick on one's car's bodywork—that are not morally wrong, even though they may reveal moral shortcomings. The objection has to be developed in some way.

The feminist critique is one way in which it is developed. Feminists have noted that women account for a disproportionate amount of cosmetic surgery patients—although the trends show that it is now much less disproportionate than it once was. More women than men seek cosmetic surgery, it is argued, because patriarchal society imposes standards of beauty and youthfulness on women that it does not impose on men. Women, it is often argued, are under much greater pressure to look young and beautiful than are men. Women are devalued if they do not conform to these standards and are thus pressured into seeking cosmetic surgery. Once some women make use of cosmetic surgery, other women are at a greater relative disadvantage and there is increased pressure on them to "go under the knife." Thus, it is argued, cosmetic surgery not only results from patriarchal standards but also entrenches and strengthens them.

Although some feminists categorically oppose cosmetic surgery (at least of the enhancement kind), others recognize that the matter is more complicated. The first complicating feature is that it may be unfair to an individual woman to condemn her for resorting to cosmetic surgery when her failure to do so leaves her at a disadvantage. Although one might bemoan the fact that she would be disadvantaged without the surgery, it is still the case that she would be disadvantaged. Is it fair to condemn her for giving herself the best chance? Second, feminists who categorically oppose cosmetic surgery face the following problem. In charging that women who consent to cosmetic surgery are but dupes of patriarchy, they run the risk of infantilizing women —of treating them as though they were children, incapable of making their own decisions. This, obviously, is an implication that feminists should want to avoid.

In their chapter in this volume, Rosemarie Tong and Hilde Lindemann, offer a feminist critique of cosmetic surgery that is not oblivious to these and other complexities. They conclude that it may sometimes be reasonable for a woman to elect to have such surgery and she should not then be condemned. Their chapter is preceded by Stephen Coleman's contribution to this book. His approach is not specifically feminist (although is also not incompatible with it), and he offers a different and more enthusiastic defense of cosmetic surgery.

## PLACEBO SURGERY

In the final chapters, David Neil and Alex London discuss the ethical problems raised by placebo surgery. The "placebo effect" is well known. Sometimes, when people are given an inert substance—a placebo[26]—that they think is a drug administered to cure or relieve the symptoms of some ailment, they actually experience some improvement in their condition. Because the placebo is inert, the effect cannot be attributable to any active agent. Instead, it must be attributable to psychological factors. The mere belief that a medicine has been administered has a medicinal effect.

The placebo effect poses a potential threat to the reliability of a clinical drug trial—one does not know to what extent the effect of the drug is attributable to the drug itself and to what extent it is attributable to the placebo effect. The standard way of countering this uncertainty is to administer a placebo rather than nothing to the control group. In this way, one controls for the placebo effect. Since all trial subjects are administered a substance, the placebo effect applies to both arms of the trial. Any net effect in the active arm must thus be over and above the placebo effect.

There are a number of obvious moral problems with placebos. First they involve some deception. One cannot experience the placebo effect if one *knows* that one is taking a placebo. This problem is addressed in clinical trials by explaining to potential research subjects that, if they enter the trial, they will be randomized blindly to either an active or placebo arm. In other words, although they will not know whether they are receiving a drug or a placebo, they do know that they may be receiving either. The second moral problem with placebos is that it would be ethically questionable to administer them—or even to ask patients to enter into a trial in which they were used—if one had good evidence that some medication were effective. Thus one condition for the use of placebos is the "equipoise" condition. Following this condition, placebos may only be administered when the evidence for whether or not the trial drug is effective is equally balanced, and when there is no other drug that is known to be an effective treatment. In such cases, the use of a placebo is justified because one really does not know if the active drug does any good and thus whether it is any better than anything else one could do, including nothing.

Placebo is as important in surgical research as it is in drug research. This is because one cannot know to what extent any improvement is the result of a patient's mere belief that the surgery is effective. Placebo surgery is more contested than placebo drugs, however, because it is more risky. Although nobody knows whether a placebo "drug" will do any good—whether it will have the placebo effect—it *is* known that it cannot do any harm. This is because it is inert. Placebo surgery, by contrast, can harm. Because the patient must not know whether he or she is undergoing the surgical procedure that is being tested or the placebo surgery, the subjective conditions of surgery must be created in the placebo case. This involves at least anesthetic and incision, and often more. Because such sham surgery, as it is also known, is still surgery, it carries the risks of surgery. For example, there can be negative reactions to the anesthetic or infection as a result of the incision.

The key question, then, is whether these risks and costs may be inflicted on research subjects, even with their consent. Sometimes the problem is presented as a clash between the interests of current research subjects and future people who will benefit from better information about which surgical interventions help and which do not. However, because placebo-controlled surgical trials have been known to show that widely accepted treatments actually are ineffective, it is far from clear that those assigned to the placebo arms are really at any disadvantage. Until we know from a placebo-controlled trial that some surgical intervention actually works, it is not at all clear that we are unfair to those who receive the placebo surgery. Because the alternative for them might be a more invasive but no more effective surgery, there may be no greater reason for worrying about administering the placebo than administering the "real" surgery.

## RECURRING THEMES

Although this book discusses a number of quite different contested surgeries, some underlying ethical questions recur in many topics. Thus, many of the surgical interventions discussed in this book, as well as many that are not discussed, can be considered as variations on common problems.

### The Limits of Paternalism

The first question concerns the appropriate limits of paternalism in decisions about whether to perform surgery on those—most notably, children—who lack the competence to decide for themselves. Paternalism, it is widely agreed, is appropriate where the best interests of the nonautonomous are served. Where disagreement arises is in determining whether some surgical intervention does or does not serve such a person's best interests. Much of the disagreement between opponents and proponents of infant male circumcision is disagreement about whether removing the foreskin helps or harms the child. Much of the disagreement about whether intersex children should be surgically assigned to one of the sexes is disagreement about whether doing so is best for these children. Those who think that conjoined twins should be separated typically do so because they take separation to be in the interests of one or both of the children, while those who oppose separation often do so because they deny separation is preferable.

Sometimes the disagreement about whether an intervention is in a child's best interests is attributable to conflicting views about what interests to consider. Are the relevant interests only medical (perhaps including psychological factors) or may they also include social and cultural considerations?

Although it would surely be wrong to act contrary to a child's best interests, at least unless there were sufficiently strong countervailing considerations, the best-interests standard is not the only relevant one. In some cases, it may turn out that we can neither recommend nor oppose a surgical intervention on the grounds of a child's best interests. That is to say, neither the surgical intervention nor its avoidance is clearly in the best interests of a child. In such cases, other factors may tip the scale in one direction or the other.

Many of those who are critical of infant circumcision, sex assignment of intersex children, and the separation of conjoined infant twins argue that unless surgery is clearly in a child's best interests, it is best to delay surgery until the children are able to decide for themselves. That is a reasonable suggestion—on the assumption that one considers whether it makes any difference when the surgery is performed, later or earlier. For example, if separation is more likely to be effective in infancy, then the benefit of a later autonomous decision has to be offset against the cost of delaying separation. There seems to be no reason to think that this calculation will always incline us either toward or against surgery in the pediatric period. It is much more likely that it will sometimes lead us in the one direction and other times in the opposite direction.

## Doubtful Autonomy

Although it is clear that young children are *not* autonomous and are thus incapable of deciding whether some contested surgery is best for them, it is not always clear whether adult patients *are* autonomous and capable of making a decision for themselves. Is the wannabe's decision to be an amputee autonomous? Is it an autonomous decision when a transsexual consents to a sex change? Feminists wonder whether women's decisions to have face-lifts, breast enhancements, and tummy-tucks are fully autonomous.

There is often a temptation among those who do not share the preferences of those who seek these surgeries to dismiss these preferences as either mad or silly. Consent to such surgery is then dismissed as nonautonomous, allowing space for a paternalistic refusal. This, however, is obviously too hasty. We cannot judge somebody as nonautonomous simply because they have different preferences from us or because they reach different conclusions. Even if it would be better if the transsexual had no desire to have genitalia of the opposite sex, if that desire cannot be eliminated, it may be best for the transsexual to have his or her sex changed. In other words, the decision to have a sex change may be entirely rational given an immutable underlying desire to be a member of the opposite sex. Similarly, even if it would be better if a woman lacked the desire for bigger breasts, breast enhancement may sometimes be the most rational decision if the desire cannot be expunged.

### The Limits of Autonomy

However, even when it is established that a decision to have surgery is autonomous, it does not follow that the surgery becomes morally unproblematic. The question then arises whether autonomy must—or even may—always be respected. Are there times when it is wrong or at least indecent to perform surgery that somebody requests? May a surgeon subject a person to the harms and risks attendant upon limb or face transplantation, even if that person desperately wants the transplant? May a surgeon perform sham surgery on research subjects who know and consent to the risks?

Some people believe that the only principle that need be invoked to settle questions of contested surgeries on competent adults is the principle of autonomy. In this view, if somebody sincerely wants the surgery, then there is no reason for the surgeon to withhold it. We should always defer to the preferences of an autonomous patient.

The problem with this view is that if taken to its logical conclusion, it would permit surgeons to transplant hearts from living donors who are willing to die so that another may live.[27] Although some may be willing to accept this implication, I suspect that most would not. Once it is conceded that an autonomous decision to have surgery does not always grant another a moral license to perform that surgery, we need to decide when it *does* create such license and when it does not. More specifically we would need to decide just how great the risk or harm has to be before it is wrong to respect an autonomous decision to assume this risk or harm. Obviously the risks of limb transplantation are nothing like the risks of living heart donation. In the latter case, the risk of death is 100 percent, whereas it is considerably smaller in the former case. Moreover, in deciding whether to harvest a heart from a living donor, the surgeon has to decide whether to take one person's life in order to save another's. In other words, the strong interests of two people have to be weighed against one another. By contrast, deciding on a limb transplant is largely about considering the interests only of the recipient in order to determine whether the surgery is or is not in his interests.[28] These differences, although they must be considered, do not settle the matter. There are some people who think that the risks and harms of limb or face transplantation, for example, are too great relative to their benefits. Others disagree.

## Normality and Disability

A further theme is the relationship between normality and disability. I use the word "normality" not in an evaluative sense to judge desirability, but rather in a statistical sense. In this sense, something is normal if it is usual, abnormal if it is unusual—if it deviates from the species norm. In this sense, intersex people and conjoined twins are abnormal. The usual assumption is that these kinds of abnormality are also disabilities in need of therapeutic intervention. This assumption, however, is a contested one. Disability rights advocates argue that disability is a "social construction" to which the fitting response is not therapy but social change.

This criticism strikes many people as odd. How, they wonder, can it be thought that intersex, for example, is a social construct? Surely the ambiguity of the genitalia, for example, is a natural rather than a social phenomenon? But this response misunderstands the objection. The objection is not a denial that intersex is a natural condition. Instead it is that this natural condition is a disability only if society is constructed in a certain way. In a society that obsesses about assigning everybody to one of two sexes, intersex people occupy a twilight zone in which they are subject to morbid curiosity and made to feel ashamed. Intersex would not be such a disability in a society that were less concerned with binary classifications of sex.

The social construction of disability becomes clearer when one considers the case of female genital cutting. In a society in which this is widely practiced, those girls and women who are *not* cut are deemed to be impure and will be ostracized and spurned as marriage partners. Ineligibility for marriage is a significant disadvantage in a traditional society, particularly for women. In this context, natural (intact) genitalia are not only abnormal but also a disability. The disability rights critique says that the fitting response is not to cut the genitals but rather to change the society.

Seen in this way, the disability rights critique seems extremely plausible. Although it also has some shortcomings, it is noteworthy that, even if we accept the critique, it would not necessarily follow that the relevant contested surgeries would always be both wrong and condemnable. This was already illustrated with reference to cosmetic surgery, but the point may now be made more generally. The problem lies in a conflict between collective action and individual interest. Collective action could facilitate societal change. If all parents stopped cutting their daughters' genitals, if all parents of intersex children let their ambiguous genitals be, if all parents of conjoined twins left them conjoined, there would be more uncut girls, more intersex people, and more conjoined people in society. This would likely lead to greater social accommodation. The problem, though, is that as long as most others are not acting collectively to bring about this change, it is not in any individual's interests to be blazing a trail. Trailblazers suffer social disadvantage and disability. It is thus hard to condemn parents who, seeking the best interests of their children, all things considered, subject them to a surgical procedure that normalizes and thus advantages them. And it is hard to condemn someone who opts for cosmetic surgery that enhances his or her appearance in a society where such surgery is widespread, given the disadvantage he or she would otherwise endure. At the same time, each individual who conforms to the norm only reinforces the trend and helps to constrain others to conform.

Given these tensions, there is a case to be made for working for societal change, not by prohibiting the contested surgical procedures but by changing minds in other ways. Although there are no easy ways to do this, the advantage of this strategy is that it aims at societal change without bringing this about by overriding reasonable autonomous responses to the unchanged society. Put another way, it is better, for example, to eradicate infibulation by changing the ideas that support it than to change the ideas that support it by eradicating infibulation. The former is more respectful of reasonable autonomous responses to dominant cultural attitudes.

This strategy has the effect of diminishing (but not obliterating) a surgeon's role in bringing about social change. This is not obviously a bad implication, because it is not at all clear that surgeons are best suited for being at the forefront of such change.

This does not imply that surgeons may proceed undaunted with the relevant contested surgeries. Even if an individual sometimes stands to gain from some such surgery, the discussions in this book show that he may not stand to gain a net benefit. Indeed, some of the contested surgeries may inflict quite serious harm, all things considered. It thus behooves surgeons and others to examine the moral status of these surgeries much more closely. The chapters in this book make a contribution to assessing critically a range of such contested surgeries.

## NOTES

1. This is discussed briefly in Rebecca J. Cook, Bernard M. Dickens, and Mahmoud F. Fathalla, *Reproductive Health and Human Rights* (Oxford: Oxford University Press, 2003), 298–304.

2. Some might argue that cosmetic surgery in general raises issues of deception—the patient falsely represents the enhancement as her natural state. I do not deny this possibility, but the deception issue is separable from rhinoplasty or breast augmentation, for example, in a way that it is not from hymen restoration. A nose job or breast enhancement can be valued independently of whether anybody takes the resultant nose or breasts to be natural. By contrast, the *whole* point of hymen restoration is to deceive.

3. This nomenclature is that of John Money and colleagues. See J. Money, R Jobaris, and G. Furth, "Apotemnophilia: Two Cases of Self-Demand Amputation as a Paraphilia," *Journal of Sex Research* 13 (1997): 114–25.

4. This term is Michael First's. See his "Desire for Amputation of a Limb: Paraphilia, Psychosis, or a New Type of Identity Disorder," *Psychological Medicine* 34 (2004): 1–10. Dr. First says that "apotemnophilia" is appropriate for those whose primary reason for wanting amputation is sexual. For those who seek amputation in order to "match their body to their identity," another term is needed; he suggests "body integrity identity disorder" (8).

5. Richard L. Bruno, "Devotees, Pretenders and Wannabes: Two Cases of Factitious Disability Disorder," *Sexuality and Disability* 15, no. 4 (1997): 243–60.

6. First, "Desire for Amputation of a Limb," 4.

7. Ibid.

8. Clare Dyer, "Surgeon Amputated Healthy Legs," *British Medical Journal* 320, no. 7231 (5 February 2000): 332.

9. These have been discussed in a few articles: Carl Elliott, "A New Way to Be Mad," *Atlantic Monthly*, December 2000, 72–84; Josephine Johnston and Carl Elliott, "Healthy Limb Amputation: Ethical and Legal Aspects," *Clinical Medicine* 2, no. 5 (September–October 2002): 431–35; Tim Bayne and Neil Levy, "Amputees by Choice: Body Integrity Identity Disorder and the Ethics of Amputation," *Journal of Applied Philosophy* 22, no. 1 (April 2005): 75–87.

10. Some forms of placebo surgery may be milder.

11. See, for example, G. C. Denniston, F. M. Hodges, and M. F. Milos, *Male and Female Circumcision: Medical, Legal and Ethical Considerations in Pediatric Practice* (New York: Kluwer, 1999).

12. See, for example, Nahid Toubia, "Female Circumcision as a Public Health Issue," *New England Journal of Medicine* 331, no. 1 (15 September 1994): 712–16; Alison T. Slack, "Female Circumcision: A Critical Appraisal," *Human Rights Quarterly* 10 (1988): 437–86; American Academy of Pediatrics, Committee on Bioethics, "Female Genital Mutilation," *Pediatrics* 102, no. 1 (July 1998): 153–56.

13. See, for example, Carla M. Obermeyer, "Female Genital Surgeries: The Known, the Unknown, and the Unknowable," *Medical Anthropology Quarterly* 13, no. 1 (1999): 79–106; Bettina Shell-Duncan and Ylva Hernlund, "Female 'Circumcision' in Africa: Dimensions of the Practice and Debates," in *Female 'Circumcision' in Africa: Culture, Controversy and Change,* ed. Bettina Shell-Duncan and Ylva Hernlund (Boulder, CO: Lynne Rienner, 2000), 1–40 (esp. 14–18); Linda Morison et al., "The Long-Term Reproductive Health Consequences of Female Genital Cutting in Rural Gambia: A Community-Based Survey," *Tropical Medicine and International Health* 6, no. 8 (August 2001): 643–53.

14. Doriane Lambelet Coleman, "The Seattle Compromise: Multicultural Sensitivity and Americanization," *Duke Law Journal* 47 (1998): 717–83; "Outrage at Doctor's Offer of 'Milder' Mutilation for Girls," *Cape Times*, 22 January 2004.

15. Sometimes an intersex person is referred to as an "intersexual," but there seems something odd about this word. Since "sexual" typically refers to the sex of orientation or behavior, "intersexual" sounds like an alternative to such terms as "heterosexual," "homosexual," and "bisexual." This would presumably make an "intersexual" somebody who is attracted to or has sex with intersex people. Yet "intersexual" refers to the sex that a person *is* rather than the sex of those to whom he or she is attracted.

16. Some people resist the use of "abnormality" in this context. I use the term in the statistical sense—to refer to a deviation from normal species functioning.

17. Deborah P. Merke and Stefan R. Bornstein, "Congenital Adrenal Hyperplasia," *Lancet* 365 (18 June 2005): 2125–36.

18. See, for example, Milton Diamond, "Pediatric Management of Ambiguous and Traumatized Genitalia," *Journal of Urology* 162 (September 1999): 1021–28.

19. Some people think that secrecy about a person's intersexuality is either a sign of or conducive to its being viewed as shameful. I find this unconvincing. Some matters are appropriately private even though not shameful. For example, there is nothing shameful in the fact that you had sex with your spouse last night, but it may still be a private matter that would be impertinent for a government employee to inquire about.

20. A unisex toilet is one that affords each individual, no matter what his or her sex, full privacy from all other people, irrespective of their sex (for more on this, see David Benatar, "Same-Sex Marriage and Sex Discrimination," *American Philosophical Association Newsletter on Philosophy and Law*, Fall 1997, 71–74). The addition of facilities for a third sex—intersexuals—would not be sufficient, given current assumptions and the wide variations among intersexuals.

21. Conjoined twins are often known colloquially as "Siamese twins" after a famous pair of 19th-century twins, Eng and Chang Bunker, who were born in Siam but spent much of their lives in the United States.

22. One recent exception is the case of Ladan and Laleh Bijani, the 29-year-old Iranian twins who sought separation and died intraoperatively at Raffles Hospital in Singapore (Wayne Arnold and Denise Grady, "Iran Twins Die Trying to Live Separate Lives," *New York Times*, 9 July 2003).

23. Alice Domurat Dreger, *One of Us: Conjoined Twins and the Future of Normal* (Cambridge, MA: Harvard University Press, 2004), 68.

24. However, legend has it that the twins Saint Cosmos and Saint Damian transplanted a leg in 348 C.E.

25. Shehan Hettiaratchy et al., "Lessons from Hand Transplantations," *Lancet* 357 (17 February 2001): 494–95.

26. *Placebo* is the Latin for "I shall be pleasing or acceptable" (Oxford Shorter English Dictionary). It is called this because a placebo pleases a patient more than it benefits him.

27. See Carl Elliott, "What's Wrong with Living Heart Transplantation?" in *A Philosophical Disease: Bioethics, Culture and Identity*, 103–20 (New York: Routledge, 1999).

28. I assume here, quite plausibly, that the limb donor is (at least cortically) dead and that the deceased either indicated consent or at least did not object to use of his or her limbs after death.

# I

# MALE CIRCUMCISION AND FEMALE GENITAL CUTTING

Between Prophylaxis and Child Abuse:
The Ethics of Neonatal Male Circumcision
*Michael Benatar and David Benatar*

The Ethics of Neonatal Male Circumcision:
Helping Parents to Decide
*Leslie Cannold*

Genital Alteration of Female Minors
*Dena S. Davis*

# 1

# Between Prophylaxis and Child Abuse: The Ethics of Neonatal Male Circumcision

## Michael Benatar and David Benatar

Routine neonatal male circumcision has been the subject of consider-able debate among medical professionals. This subject, however, has received negligible attention in the bioethics literature. This suggests that most scholars working in bioethics do not consider neonatal male circum-cision, unlike the practices of female genital excision that are common in parts of Africa and elsewhere, to be a morally troubling surgical proce-dure.[1] This attitude toward neonatal male circumcision seems to be shared by many people, even in societies where male circumcision is performed infrequently. That is to say, relatively few people think that the practice is morally unacceptable, even if they themselves would not have their sons circumcised.

But there are some people who *do* consider routine circumcision of chil-dren (who are too young to consent) to be morally wrong or at least morally suspect. They take circumcision to be a severely injurious prac-tice. For many of them any routine alteration of infant genitalia is a form a child abuse. By contrast, the advocates of *routine* neonatal circumcision believe that there are significant health advantages to circumcision and that these unequivocally override the costs and risks, which they believe are negligible. Although these are polar views, they are not infrequently expressed. We believe that both views are mistaken and we shall argue to this effect.

Circumcision, the removal of the foreskin, can be performed at any age and for a variety of reasons. However, we shall focus primarily on circumcision of

Reprinted, with the permission of Taylor & Francis, Inc., from the *American Journal of Bioethics*, vol. 3, no. 2 (Spring 2003), pp. 35–48.

minors for nontherapeutic purposes. An adult's decision to undergo circumcision is uncontroversial. Even the most ardent opponents of circumcision have no opposition to an autonomous adult's choosing to be circumcised.[2] Similarly uncontroversial is therapeutic (rather than allegedly prophylactic) circumcision. As most nontherapeutic circumcision is performed in the neonatal period, it is circumcision in this period that will be our primary focus, although much of our discussion will also be relevant to the circumcision of older children.

Most of those writing on the topic say that they would like parents to be able to make an informed decision about whether to have their sons circumcised. However, it is extremely difficult for those who have not immersed themselves in the literature on this topic to be able to make an informed judgment. This is, in part, because of the vastly differing interpretations of the evidence offered by different reviewers. The issues are further clouded by the use of emotive language by a number of authors, especially among those opposed to circumcision.[3] We cannot hope to review everything that has been written on the topic. Nor can we comment on the methodology and quality of every study. We shall certainly not be offering new empirical evidence. What we do plan to do, however, is to clarify some conceptual issues, something which is often neglected in the debate about circumcision. We shall also offer what we hope is a balanced outline of the evidence, before suggesting how it might reasonably be interpreted.

## MUTILATION

Those who believe that circumcision of minors is morally prohibited, often suggest that removing the foreskin constitutes mutilation of a child. For instance, George Denniston, Frederick Hodges, and Marilyn Milos note[4] that *Stedman's Medical Dictionary* defines *mutilation* as "[d]isfigurement or injury by removal or destruction of any conspicuous or essential part of the body." Male circumcision, they say, is the injurious and appearance-altering removal of a conspicuous body part and thus unquestionably constitutes mutilation. But this sort of argument begs the question. It assumes that circumcision disfigures and injures. Yet this is exactly what is in dispute in debates about whether circumcision constitutes mutilation.

This can be seen if we consider other surgical procedures such as breast reduction, liposuction, and rhinoplasty. These are all procedures that alter the appearance of parts of a person. Those who request such procedures do not take them to be disfiguring. Similarly, those who circumcise their sons do not take removal of the foreskin to be disfiguring. Even if people can be mistaken about what constitutes disfigurement, it is still true that one cannot assume that a surgical procedure is disfiguring simply because it alters the body. It may be enhancing or it may be (aesthetically) neutral—neither disfiguring nor enhancing.

Of course, even nondisfiguring surgical procedures can be injurious. Again, however, not every surgical procedure, even one that removes healthy tissue, can be assumed to be injurious. That a surgical procedure is harmful is something that must be demonstrated rather than merely asserted.

It is also possible for a disfiguring surgical procedure, all things considered, to be beneficial rather than injurious. For instance, amputating a gangrenous leg is considered by most people to be disfiguring. Such people could term it a mutilation. However, if amputation were the only way to save a person's life, it would usually be beneficial. Where a mutilation is, all things considered, a benefit, it can be morally justifiable. Thus even if circumcision is a mutilation, it does not inevitably follow that it is morally unacceptable. Further argument would be required to establish that conclusion. Although nobody would suggest that circumcision can save a life as directly as can amputation of a gangrenous leg, it is also the case that circumcision, if a disfigurement at all, is a much less radical disfigurement than a limb amputation. The benefit it would have to produce in order to be justified would thus need to be much smaller.

In short then, whether circumcision is a mutilation and, if it is, whether it is an unacceptable mutilation can be established only by argument and not by mere assumption. Potential harms and benefits must be examined and weighed against one another. This stands in contrast to the view of some opponents of circumcision who, though they believe circumcision to be harmful, say that they would still be opposed to circumcision even if it were not.[5] They take the mere removal of healthy tissue from a child to be sufficient grounds for condemning all nontherapeutic circumcision of boys.[6] But the ethics of a surgical procedure cannot be assessed independently of whatever harms and benefits it does or does not have. To think that a moral judgment can be made without considering these is to adopt what sounds like a dogma, rather than a reasoned conclusion.

## INFORMED CONSENT

One reason why some opponents of circumcision think that circumcision can be condemned without considering what harms or benefits it may have is that they think appropriate consent cannot be obtained. Children, they correctly note, lack the capacity to consent to circumcision. It is usually parents who provide consent for the circumcision of their children. However, those opposed to any nontherapeutic circumcision of minors claim that parents are entitled to consent to surgical procedures for their children only when there is immediate and clear medical necessity.[7] Accordingly, they regard circumcision of children to be a form of assault—which is what surgery amounts to when appropriate consent or exceptional circumstances (such as necessity) are absent.

But is it really true that parents are morally entitled to authorize medical interventions, only for clear and immediate medical necessity? In parts of the world where diseases against which children are often vaccinated are now uncommon, the necessity of such vaccination for any individual child is neither clear[8] nor immediate. Moreover, there are very small but real risks (including death) from vaccination. A child's informed consent for such vaccination cannot be obtained. The choice (where government allows a choice rather than simply requiring universal inoculation) can thus either be deferred to proxy decision makers such as the parents or left to the adult that the child will become. But delaying vaccination can undermine much of its benefit. It thus seems entirely reasonable that parents or other guardians of a child's best interests be morally entitled to decide for the child. The role of a parent is not simply to save children from immediate catastrophe, but to protect and foster a child's long-term best interests. That is why most people think that parents may consent on behalf of their children not only to vaccination but also to such procedures as orthodontics and various nonmedical interventions including schooling.

There are limits, of course, on the sorts of things to which parents can consent on behalf of their children. Typically the things to which parents may not consent are those which are unequivocally harmful to their children. Perhaps those opposed to circumcision believe that it is just such a procedure. That, however, is a much stronger claim than the claim that circumcision is not a clear and immediate medical necessity, and it is accordingly much harder to defend. Nor can it be argued that there is nothing to be lost by delaying a choice about circumcision of one's child until he can make it himself. This is because there are costs to delaying circumcision until adulthood. At the very least, circumcision may be psychologically unpleasant in adults in a way that it is not in infants. Moreover, the risks are greater in adults. Finally, although, as we shall show, the evidence for beneficial effects of circumcision is controversial, insofar as there are these benefits, they are significantly reduced if the circumcision is performed later in life.

## ALLEGED COSTS AND BENEFITS

Having established that a moral assessment of neonatal circumcision cannot be made without considering whatever costs and benefits it may have, we turn now to the empirical evidence about these matters. We shall examine each issue individually to determine whether there is a cost or a benefit and, if so, its magnitude. After we have considered each of these issues, we shall attempt to draw an overall conclusion about the net medical value of neonatal circumcision.

## Pain

A compelling objection to neonatal circumcision is that it has usually been practiced without any anaesthesia.[9] It is now well known that neonates are capable
of feeling pain[10] and it is widely accepted that neonatal circumcision is a painful
procedure. This recognition has led to a search for suitable analgesia. Among
the techniques that have been employed are topical analgesia with EMLA
cream, dorsal penile nerve block, and ring block. In randomised controlled
trials, the topical cream has been shown to be effective in reducing the pain
response[11] but not as effective as the two nerve block techniques.[12] The high
efficacy of dorsal penile nerve block has been repeatedly demonstrated in
neonates.[13] Studies in adults have shown that either ring block or dorsal penile
nerve block combined with anaesthesia of the frenulum are more often effective than dorsal penile nerve block alone.[14] The limited use of regional anaesthesia is attributable to misperceptions that the procedure is difficult to perform, that it carries significant risks, and that it causes more pain than the
circumcision itself. In fact, the analgesia can be administered with ease.
Although minor complications such as limited bruising have commonly been
observed, these healed spontaneously[15] and complications of any clinical significance are rare.[16] Finally, the administration of the injections themselves have
not been found to elicit a pain response.[17]

Even if adequate analgesia is provided for the procedure itself, concern
might be raised about postoperative pain. We are not aware of any studies
on such pain and its control in neonates. There seems to be no reason, however, why simple topical or systemic analgesics should not suffice. Therefore,
concerns about postoperative pain cannot constitute strong grounds against
performing the procedure.

## Complications

As with any surgical procedure, circumcision carries a risk of complications,
including most commonly bleeding and sepsis. Studies that have looked at
large numbers of children who were circumcised, have reported varying
rates of complications from 0.06 percent[18] to 55 percent.[19] This apparent dis-
crepancy is attributable to the definition of *complication* that is employed.
Those studies that report high complication rates have included even minor
post-procedure oozing of blood from the wound. That interpretation, however, is unreasonably broad and is inconsistent with what would constitute
a complication in any other surgical procedure. The consensus, even
among those reporting high complication rates, is that the incidence of clinically significant complications is very low. It is commonly thought to
be around 0.19 percent to 1.5 percent.[20] It is also agreed that even where
there are complications, the majority of these either resolve spontaneously
or are easily resolved by simple medical intervention. There are, of course,

instances of more severe complications, as described in some case reports. These can include denuded penile shaft, laceration or necrosis of the glans, urethral fistula, and death. However, these are very uncommon. The risk of death, for example is less than 1 per 500,000.[21]

## Penile Cancer

It has often been claimed that circumcision is protective against penile cancer. A simplistic approach to this issue is to compare the incidence of the disease in societies where circumcision is widely practiced with its incidence in societies where only a minority of males are circumcised. Both advocates and opponents of neonatal circumcision have adopted this approach in (partial) support of their respective views. Opponents of circumcision, for instance, have noted that the incidence of penile cancer in the United States, where the vast majority of males are circumcised, is *higher* (0.9–1.0 per 100,000 males) than in Denmark (0.82 per 100,000 males) where circumcision is extremely uncommon.[22] By contrast, proponents of routine circumcision cite the extremely low incidence of penile cancer in Israel (0.1 per 100,000 males),[23] where circumcision is even more prevalent than in the United States.[24]

This is a very indirect approach to the issue. It (1) determines the incidence of a disease in two populations; (2) notes the prevalence of circumcision in these populations; and then (3) makes an inference about the relationship between the disease and circumcision status. It is indirect because it does not actually determine whether patients with the disease are circumcised.

There are studies that have adopted a more direct approach. They have examined patients with penile cancer and established what proportion of them are circumcised. These include studies of penile cancer in New York (120 cases),[25] Illinois (139 cases),[26] New York (100 cases),[27] and Michigan (156 cases).[28] None of these 515 patients were neonatally circumcised. One concern with these studies is that the investigators did not control for possible confounding variables, which might include smoking, sexual behavior, socioeconomic status, and sexually transmitted diseases. Nevertheless, the overwhelming nature of the results suggests that they cannot therefore be dismissed. More recent studies have attempted to control for potential confounding factors. For instance, a study of 110 penile cancer patients (and 355 controls) in Washington state and the province of British Columbia found that, although other factors may also increase the risk of penile cancer, not being circumcised neonatally carried a 3.2 times greater risk for the development of this disease.[29]

Other recent studies have been even more refined, not only controlling for potentially confounding variables, but also distinguishing between various forms of (squamous cell) penile cancer. The results of studies that make this distinction suggest that circumcision is protective against the more but not less severe forms of this disease. The spectrum of diseases that can be included under this rubric ranges, in increasing order of severity, from penile intraepithelial neoplasia (PIN) to carcinoma in situ (CIS) to invasive penile carcinoma (IPC). A study published in 1993 from the Mayo Clinic in Minnesota of 34 patients with penile cancer found that although low-grade PIN occurred in the 12 neonatally circumcised men, all the cases of CIS and IPC occurred in men who were not circumcised in infancy.[30] In an even more recent study of 213 penile cancer patients in California, in which the circumcision status was known in 207 of them, 84.3 percent of the CIS and 97.7 percent of the IPC patients were not neonatally circumcised.[31]

None of these studies can be regarded as ideal or definitive. Among some of their potential shortcomings are their retrospective nature, small sample size, and use of self-report as a means of determining circumcision status.[32] Nevertheless, the preponderance of evidence suggests that neonatal circumcision is protective against (or at least associated with a lower incidence of) the more severe forms of penile cancer.[33] Given that it is the more severe forms of this disease that entail greater morbidity and mortality, preventing these is of greater benefit.

We are not claiming that penile cancer, or even its more severe forms, does not occur in men who were neonatally circumcised. Nor do we wish to enter into the (distracting) protracted debate about exactly how many cases (or case reports) of penile cancer there have been in U.S. men circumcised in infancy. Some proponents of circumcision have claimed that there have been only 10 such case reports within the last 55 years.[34] Opponents of circumcision have criticised this claim at great length,[35] citing a few additional case reports and noting that not every case will have been reported in the medical literature. While there may be technical validity to at least some of these criticisms, they fail to get to the heart of the issue. It is inadequate to cite a few case reports in response to the numerous sizeable case series that have shown that the overwhelming majority of cases of invasive penile cancer occur in men who were not circumcised in infancy.[36]

## Urinary Tract Infection

The relationship between urinary tract infection (UTI) and circumcision has been the subject of many studies and the consensus in the medical literature is that circumcision is associated with a lower incidence of UTI.[37] We are aware of no studies that have shown either the reverse or no association. Lower incidence of UTI is one of the benefits most commonly cited in support of circumcision.[38]

That said, it must be emphasized, however, that there *is* disagreement about the magnitude of the increased risk of UTI among uncircumcised boys. Some studies have reported a 3.7-fold[39] increased risk of UTI in uncircumcised compared with circumcised children. Others have suggested as much as a 12-fold[40] increase.

There have been criticisms of the methodology of these studies. These include most of the studies' retrospective nature, the inclusion of primarily only hospitalized patients, and the failure to control adequately for confounding variables (such as socioeconomic factors). All these are legitimate concerns and do show ways in which the studies have not been ideal. However, it is not reasonable, for these reasons, to completely disregard these data. First, one cannot ignore that, despite the varying limitations of the numerous studies, all have pointed in the same direction. Second, not all available medical evidence conforms to the highest standards and it is necessary to base practice on the available evidence, which, although defective, is not so thoroughly flawed as to be entirely useless. Medical evidence does vary in its quality and, if one were to reject all evidence that was less than ideal, one would be left with no basis for decision making in many areas of medical practice, not to mention everyday life.

Having established that there is an increased risk of UTI among uncircumcised boys, the significance of this needs to be assessed. Here, some advocates of circumcision have tended to overrate the value of circumcision. Any fair assessment of its significance must consider the following. While it is true that circumcision confers a 10-fold risk reduction of UTI, the absolute incidence of UTI is low, with 0.15 percent of circumcised and 1.5 percent of uncircumcised male infants developing such an infection. Put another way, UTI does not occur in 99.85 percent of circumcised infant males and in 98.5 percent of uncircumcised infant boys. Moreover, most UTIs occur in the first year of life and are easily diagnosed and treatable, with low morbidity and mortality. More serious complications of UTI, such as vesico-ureteric reflux, renal scarring, pylonephritis, and renal failure are possible but occur with low frequency.[41] In summary then, circumcision does seem to confer a small but real benefit in terms of UTI prevention.

## Sexually Transmitted Diseases

Circumcision has also been claimed to be protective against some sexually transmitted diseases (STDs), including human immunodeficiency virus (HIV). Although the evidence for this claim is not unproblematic, the data on HIV is more consistent than that on other STDs. Furthermore, given the availability of a number of systematic reviews as well as a recent meta-analysis on HIV and circumcision status, the data on HIV is easier to assess. For this reason, we shall discuss HIV and non-HIV STDs separately. We shall first consider the latter.

### STDs Other Than HIV

*Genital ulcer disease* (GUD) is one category of STD. Of the five studies that looked at syphilis, four reported reduced risk in those who are circumcised[42] and one reported no difference.[43] Herpes was investigated in six studies. Three concluded that circumcised men have a reduced risk[44] and three found no difference.[45] One study of chancroid (*Haemophilus ducreyi*) found that circumcised men were less susceptible.[46] Two studies examined genital ulcer disease without specifying the infecting organism and both similarly found reduced risk in circumcised men.[47]

Consider next the studies that examined *urethritis*. Of these, gonorrhoea was the subject of investigation in seven studies. Three concluded that circumcised men were at less risk[48] and four found no significant difference.[49] Six studies considered non-gonoccocal urethritis (NGU). Two found circumcised men to be at increased risk[50] and four found no significant difference.[51]

Four of the studies investigated *genital warts*. Circumcised men were found to be at increased risk in two.[52] Two studies found no difference in the risk faced by circumcised and uncircumcised men.[53]

Robert Van Howe, a well-known opponent of circumcision, judges on the basis of this and other data, that "no solid epidemiological evidence has been found to support the theory that circumcision prevents STDs."[54] In his view the "only consistent trend is that uncircumcised males may be more susceptible to GUD, while circumcised men are more prone to urethritis."[55]

Over the years, the American Academy of Pediatrics has issued a number of position statements about neonatal circumcision. The most recent of these, which was published in 1999,[56] had very little to say about STDs. They concluded that "circumcised males may be less at risk for syphilis than are uncircumcised males."[57] Others have been more enthusiastic about the protection circumcision affords against STDs. Edgar Schoen, a well-known defender of routine neonatal circumcision, and his colleagues, state that "[s]trong evidence . . . links lack of male circumcision to increased risk for genital ulcer disease, particularly chancroid and syphilis."[58] Stephen Moses and his colleagues, in reviewing a host of studies, claim that "there is good concordance for an association between lack of circumcision with chancroid, syphilis, genital herpes, and gonorrhoea. Only for urethritis other than gonorrhoea and genital warts is the evidence for an effect of circumcision inconclusive."[59]

## Human Immunodeficiency Virus

Evaluating the claim that circumcision is associated with a lower incidence of HIV infection[60] is greatly facilitated by a number of *systematic* reviews as well as a meta-analysis. Stephen Moses and his colleagues reviewed thirty studies.[61] Twenty-two of these (including two prospective studies) found a statistically significant association between lack of circumcision and HIV infection. (The magnitude of the increased risk for the uncircumcised ranged from 1.5 to 8.4.) Four studies in the review found a trend toward an association and four studies found no association.

More recently, Helen Weiss and colleagues performed a meta-analysis of 28 published studies that evaluated the risk factors for susceptibility to HIV-1 infection in men in sub-Saharan Africa.[62] In 21 studies, circumcision was associated with a reduced risk of HIV infection, the difference being statistically significant in 14. A higher risk of HIV infection in circumcised men was observed in 6 studies (4 from a single area) but none reached statistical significance. Overall, circumcision was associated with a highly significant reduction in the risk of HIV infection (RR = 0.52). Significant heterogeneity was observed between the studies, indicating that the magnitude of the protective effect varied in different populations, with the association between circumcision and susceptibility to HIV infection being strongest in high-risk patients.

Robert Van Howe reviewed and analyzed 33 studies.[63] He concluded that circumcision is associated with an *increased* risk of acquiring and transmitting HIV. However, Stephen Moses and colleagues have raised some powerful objections to this study.[64] They have pointed to and explained the methodological flaw of combining raw data for re-analysis, as Robert Van Howe does. That this analysis is flawed stands to reason when one compares the results of the individual studies cited by Dr. Van Howe with the conclusions he reaches via his analysis. Of the 33 studies he examined, 16 showed an association between lack of circumcision and increased risk of HIV infection, 4 suggested a trend toward this association, 12 demonstrated no association and only 1 showed an increased risk of HIV among circumcised men. Nigel O'Farrell and Matthias Egger[65] have pointed to the same methodological flaws in Robert Van Howe's analysis. Moreover, they have reanalyzed the studies he reviewed and, in contrast to him, they concluded that lack of circumcision is associated with an increased risk of HIV infection. They note that this relationship is only present in groups at high risk for HIV infection.

### Reliability of the Primary Data

Numerous objections have been raised against the primary studies on the relationship between circumcision status and sexually transmitted diseases. One problem is that of publication bias—that there is a tendency not to submit or to publish studies which suggest no effect. This is a genuine concern, not only with regard to this issue, but with the whole enterprise of scientific publication. Nevertheless, one is only able to base judgments on available evidence. Other, more important problems, are those of selection bias (how individuals are identified for inclusion in the study), the method of ascertaining circumcision status, the type of study (whether prospective, retrospective, etc.), and the degree to which confounding variables are controlled. While individual studies may be subject to criticism on some or other of these grounds, it is also the case that many primary studies have avoided these pitfalls to varying extents and nonetheless found circumcision associated with lower risk of STDs including HIV. The review by Stephen Moses and his colleagues,[66] for example, included two population-based studies as well as two prospective studies. On the issue of determining a subject's circumcision status, Helen Weiss and her coauthors excluded from their analysis those primary studies that used a proxy (such as religion) for circumcision,[67] and many studies have used doctor examination rather than self-report.[68] Many studies controlled for confounding variables. Robert Bailey and colleagues found that even controlling for differences in sexual practices and hygienic behavior, circumcised men were at lower risk.[69] In their meta-analysis, for example, Helen Weiss and colleagues noted that some adjustment for confounding factors was reported in 15 of 21 studies regarding HIV.[70] Among the factors controlled for were age, ethnic group, marital status, area of residence, sexual behavior, and condom use. Although the controlling for confounding variables is much better in the HIV studies, there are some studies on non-HIV STDs that controlled for confounding variables, such as age, ethnicity, marital status, and number of sexual partners.[71]

What the above shows, we believe, is that the evidence is stronger and of a better quality for HIV (particularly in high-risk heterosexual groups) than for other STDs, and that it is stronger for some non-HIV STDs than for others. Although none of the evidence is anywhere near conclusive, it also cannot be ignored. The criticisms of the studies that have been done, although having a certain force, are insufficient to discard those studies and their findings.

## Other Considerations

There are a number of other issues that are raised in debates about the medical value or risks of circumcision. For instance, circumcision has been claimed to facilitate genital hygiene. This claim is false under some interpretations and true under others. It is not the case that maintaining genital hygiene is very difficult for an uncircumcised man. However, it is the case that it takes slightly more effort than for a circumcised man. That slight difference is not important in itself, but it would be somewhat significant if uncircumcised men, either in the absence of or contrary to any attempts at education about genital hygiene, tended not to exert that extra effort. Unfortunately, there is simply very little and uncompelling data on the basis of which any judgment about this matter can be made.[72]

Circumcision has also been said to protect against phimosis[73] and paraphimosis.[74] Although these conditions can only occur in those who are uncircumcised (or incompletely circumcised), their incidence is very low.[75] Thus circumcision, where it is not incompletely done, does prevent these conditions in the small proportion of men who would otherwise have acquired either of them. It has also been claimed that balanitis[76] is more common in the uncircumcised. Nevertheless, the incidence remains low.[77]

Meatitis[78] and meatal ulceration occur more often in the circumcised.[79] There are only a few studies that bear on these issues, and those that do are old. Thus caution is required in the conclusions one draws from this data.

There have been some suggestions that there is a lower incidence of cervical cancer in the female partners of circumcised men. However, there is widespread agreement that there is inadequate data to make such a claim.[80]

Finally, conflicting claims have been made about the relationship between circumcision and sexual pleasure in the man and his female partner. On the one hand, it has been argued that circumcised men experience less sexual pleasure. This has been explained by the keratinization of the exposed glans and the loss of the highly erogenous preputial tissue. However, what little evidence there is on this matter suggests that the circumcised glans is no less sensitive.[81] Moreover, removal of erogenous tissue does not necessarily entail diminished sexual pleasure if sufficient erogenous tissue remains. Others have argued that sexual dysfunction is less common in circumcised men[82] and that the circumcised status is preferred by female partners. Sexual preferences for the circumcised or uncircumcised state will depend on many variables, including culture. It thus seems ill advised to draw general conclusions from the very few studies there have been.

## WEIGHING UP COSTS AND BENEFITS

It should be clear from our surveying of the available evidence about circumcision that the practice has both costs and benefits. The most significant cost of neonatal circumcision is the pain that accompanies it. Performing this procedure without adequate analgesia, as is usually the case, is of great moral concern. Given that safe and effective local anaesthesia for neonatal circumcision is possible, there is no excuse for failing to use it. Where it is used, this major cost can be eliminated or at least significantly reduced. While there can be complications from circumcision, these are mostly minor. Clinically significant negative sequelae are extremely rare. The available evidence suggests that circumcision is protective against the more severe forms of penile cancer and has a small but real effect in reducing the incidence of urinary tract infections. Circumcision is also associated with a lower risk of genital ulcer disease, but a slightly increased risk of urethritis. At least in high-risk heterosexual groups, circumcision also seems to lower susceptibility to HIV infection.

This would suggest that the potential benefits of neonatal circumcision slightly outweigh the costs, although this is not obviously so. There are a few reasons for being cautious about judging that the balance tips in favor of circumcision. First, the data is incomplete. For instance, the true incidence of serious complications is unknown. Second, not every potential cost and benefit will be equally relevant in every circumstance. For instance, in communities where the incidence of penile cancer and sexually transmitted diseases is very low, the expected benefits of circumcision will be far fewer than in societies in which these conditions are more prevalent. Finally, an overall assessment of the medical costs and benefits of circumcision cannot be made independent of personal value judgments. For example, different people will make different judgments regarding whether reducing the small risk of penile cancer is worth the remote risk of a serious complication from circumcision.

For these reasons, we think that neonatal circumcision cannot unequivocally be said to yield a net medical gain or loss. In other words, it is not something that can be said to be routinely indicated, nor something that is routinely contraindicated. It is a discretionary matter. The decision whether or not to circumcise a child should thus be made by the parents, who, within certain limits, are entitled to employ their own value judgments in furtherance of their child's best interests. These limits are not exceeded in most decisions about neonatal circumcision, given the nature of the medical evidence.

## CULTURE

Prior to the last century, it was not medical, but rather cultural and religious reasons for which circumcision was most often performed. Circumcision continues to be practiced for such reasons by many people. Cultural practices do not have trumping moral weight. That is to say, simply because a practice is culturally valued does not mean that it is morally acceptable. Sometimes a culture treats people in such harmful ways that these people's rights are violated. The practices of widow burning and foot binding are examples. Were it the case that male circumcision unequivocally inflicted as serious harms as do these practices, then its cultural value would be morally overridden. However, the available medical evidence does not support this conclusion and thus such a consideration cannot outweigh the powerful cultural value that circumcision has for many people. Two papers that performed a formal cost-benefit analysis of neonatal male circumcision also reached the conclusion, given the nature of the medical evidence, that cultural and religious considerations should determine whether circumcision is performed.[83]

This is not to say that people should accept their cultural practices uncritically, even if the weight of evidence does not speak against them. It is all too easy (and common) to privilege those cultural ways to which one is accustomed on account of their familiarity. There is a value in stepping back from one's cultural assumptions. When one does that regarding male circumcision, or if one views this practice from another cultural perspective, one can only wonder what possessed ancient people to first think of removing the foreskin. Considered independently, it is about as strange as deciding to re-move a part of the earlobe from all children.

This is just the view many people have of clitoridectomy, for example. Of course, this practice, in addition to being strange, is also very harmful. It is this harm that separates female genital excision from male circumcision. Neverthe-less the inability of many people to step back from their cultural unfamiliarity with genital alterations of young girls, is reflected in discussions about how Western societies should relate to female genital excision either in their coun-tries of origin or where immigrants wish to bring the practice to their new Western homes. In such discussions, the usual line of argument is that the prac-tice should be entirely eliminated rather than modified to make it less harmful and more akin to male circumcision. More specifically, it is suggested that it would be an unacceptable strategy to encourage a less damaging form of gen-ital surgery as a way of accommodating cultural ways while minimizing their harmfulness. Excision of the clitoral prepuce is anatomically neither more nor less radical a procedure than removal of the penile foreskin.[84] Yet, many of those who would not think twice about circumcising a boy would balk at per-mitting even the partial removal of a young girl's prepuce.

Some might explain their antipathy only to the latter by arguing that the removal of female genital tissue is historically rooted in misogynistic ideas because the expressed aim of female genital cutting is often to curb female sexuality. This, the opponents of the practice may say, oppresses women. Thus the fitting response is not to refine the practice but to abolish it. But this explanation reflects the very cultural bias to which we have referred, be-cause it is far from clear that there is an asymmetry here between the re-moval of analogous bits of male and female genital tissue. Consider the fol-lowing three possibilities. (1) If removing the preputial tissue curbs sexuality of both sexes and if, on the basis of curbing female sexuality, the removal of the female prepuce is misogynistic, then the removal of the male foreskin should be viewed as misandristic. (2) If removing preputial tissue curbs sex-uality but male circumcision is not misandristic because it also affirms the male in the eyes of the community, then female circumcision, which also af-firms females in their communities, is not misogynistic. Finally, (3) if remov-ing preputial tissue does not curb sexuality in either sex, then the basis for saying that the removal of the clitoral prepuce is misogynistic is eliminated.

The culturally blinded person fails to see that just as female circumcision has been judged, both by its supporters and its opponents, to curb female sexuality, so has male circumcision been said, again by both its supporters and detractors, to curb male sexuality.[85] And they fail to see that just as male circumcision is seen (often simultaneously) as an affirmation of the male, so female circumcision is seen (often simultaneously) as an affirmation of the female. While the removal of the clitoris and labia is indeed clearly unlike the removal of the male foreskin, the same cannot be said of the removal of analogous tissues.

There are other differences, of course, between the removal of male and female preputial tissue. For instance, although there is some evidence about the medical value of male circumcision there is none about a comparable benefit in females. There are two possible explanations for this: (1) that the female procedure has no medical benefits; or (2) that there may be such benefits but the matter has not received any scientific attention (yet). However, we suspect that the opposition to excising the clitoral prepuce is based not so much on the absence of medical evidence for a benefit, as on an abhorrence for removing genital tissue from a girl.[86] This suggests an asymmetrical judgment about the intrinsic acceptability of removing preputial tissue. This asymmetry can be addressed either by extending the rejection of genital alteration to male circumcision or by withdrawing it from the comparable procedure in females. Until symmetrical judgments are made about comparable procedures, we have every reason to believe that our cultural assumptions are blinding us one way or the other.

We are not endorsing or condemning cultural views in favor of or against (non-harmful) circumcision. We are suggesting that there are cultural biases and that comparable practices (if they really are comparable) should be weighted equally. We are also suggesting that cultural views can themselves be subject to scrutiny and evaluation, and one way this can be done is by reflecting on analogous practices in other cultures to determine whether one's cultural views are consistent.

## THE BURDEN OF PROOF

It may be objected that our argument for the moral acceptability of circumcision rests on a mistaken presumption about when elective surgery[87] is permissible. More specifically, it might be said that it is not the mere absence of harm that renders surgery permissible, but also the presence of clear and significant net benefit. In other words, it might be argued, it is not sufficient to show that a surgical intervention will not be harmful. There must, in addition, be a demonstrable benefit. However, if we are correct that there are no clear and significant *medical* benefits to be derived from circumcision, there may still be *other* kinds of benefits.[88] Thus the crucial question is whether the relevant presumption should be that (1) surgery is impermissible unless it offers clear and significant net *medical* benefit; or (2) surgery is impermissible unless it offers clear and significant net (medical or nonmedical) benefit. Those who would opt for the first presumption would have to explain why it is that medical benefits are the only relevant ones. It is not as though medical benefits are necessarily or always more important. Some medical benefits are minor and some nonmedical benefits are of great importance. There seems no reason to privilege the one kind of benefit over the other, simply because the one is a medical benefit. Nor is it clear why medicine should be used to secure only some kinds of benefits.

If education, for example, may be used for medical or cultural benefit and if engineering may be used for social benefit, why may medicine not be used (within appropriate limits) for cultural or other human benefit? There is obviously much more that can be said about this issue. However, resolving this issue would take us well beyond a focus on circumcision to a host of other less or uncontested practices, which space constraints prevent.

## CONCLUSION

We have examined both conceptual issues and empirical evidence pertaining to neonatal circumcision of boys. Our conclusion is that circumcision is neither a compelling prophylactic measure nor a form of child abuse. For this reason, nontherapeutic circumcision of infant boys is a suitable matter for parental discretion. In exercising that discretion, religious and cultural factors, though preferably subject to critical evaluation, may reasonably play a role. That our conclusion occupies the popular middle ground between those who condemn the practice outright and those who think it should be routinely performed, does not provide grounds for accepting it. The middle way is sometimes the wrong way. In the circumcision debate, however, the evidence and arguments support neither of the extremes.

## NOTES

This article is the product of a close collaborative effort, with each author contributing equally, but in different ways. Although both authors worked on all aspects of the paper together, Michael Benatar was primarily responsible for interpreting the medical evidence and David Benatar bore primary responsibility for the ethical analysis.

1. There are some exceptions. See, for example, Margaret A. Somerville, "Respect in the context of infant male circumcision: can ethics and law provide insights?" in George C. Denniston, Frederick Mansfield Hodges and Marilyn Fayre Milos (Eds.), *Male and Female Circumcision: Medical Legal and Ethical Considerations in Pediatric Practice*, New York: Kluwer, 1999; 413–24.

2. Opposition to circumcision of even a consenting adult is a conceivable view, but it is not one we have heard expressed.

3. One pair of authors, in speaking about proponents of circumcision remarked: "We sincerely hope that they are more interested in preventing penile cancer than in perpetrating unethical, destructive, mutilative, antisexual, Bronze Age blood rituals on defenceless children" [Paul M. Fleiss and Frederick Hodges, "Neonatal circumcision and penile cancer—authors' reply," *British Medical Journal* 1996; 313; 47]. Others referred to an infant's response to circumcision as ". . . screams of *agony* and *protest* . . ." (our emphasis) [George C. Denniston, "Tyranny of the Victims: An analysis of Circumcision Advocacy," in George C. Denniston, Frederick Mansfield Hodges and Marilyn Fayre Milos (Eds.), *Male and Female Circumcision: Medical Legal and Ethical Considerations in Pediatric Practice*, New York: Kluwer, 1999, p. 223].

4. George C. Denniston, Frederick Mansfield Hodges and Marilyn Fayre Milos, "Preface" in George C. Denniston, Frederick Mansfield Hodges and Marilyn Fayre Milos (Eds.), *Male and Fe-*

*male Circumcision: Medical Legal and Ethical Considerations in Pediatric Practice*, New York: Kluwer, 1999, pp. vi–vii.

5. Ibid, p. v.

6. Ibid.

7. Ibid, p. vi; Robert S. Van Howe, "Response to 'Determinants of Decision Making for Circumcision' by C. Ciesielski-Carlucci, N. Milliken and N. H. Cohen (*CQ*, Vol. 5, No. 2)," *Cambridge Quarterly of Healthcare Ethics*, 1997; 6: 88–89, 88.

8. When an infectious disease is uncommon in a particular population, the individual benefits from widespread vaccination that results in herd immunity. It is not clear, however, that the individual benefits from his own vaccination in the context of herd immunity.

9. A sucrose nipple and, in Jewish ritual circumcision, a few drops of wine, have been used, but these do not constitute proper analgesia.

10. K. J. S. Anand and P. R. Hickey, "Pain and its effects in the human neonate and fetus," *New England Journal of Medicine*, 1987; 317(21): 1321–29. This paper has been widely cited, including by numerous other studies that have investigated the question of neonatal (and late fetal) pain. That neonates can feel pain is accepted by almost everybody. Stuart Derbyshire is an isolated dissenter. ["Locating the beginnings of pain," *Bioethics*, 1999; 13(1): 1–31.] We have demonstrated ["A pain in the fetus: toward ending confusion about fetal pain," *Bioethics*, 2001; 15(1): 57–76] how he misrepresents the scientific consensus, employs a confused and narrow interpretation of the concept of pain, and reaches a conclusion which is not supported by the available evidence. In his attempt to respond to our paper ["Fetal pain: an infantile debate," *Bioethics*, 2001; 15(1): 77–84] he does not engage our criticisms and simply repeats his earlier errors (this time with invective).

11. Franca Benini, Celeste Johnston, Daniel Faucher and J. V. Aranda, "Topical anesthesia during circumcision in newborn infants," *JAMA*, 1993; 270(7): 850–53.

12. Janice Lander, Barbara Brady-Fryer, James B. Metcalfe, Shemin Nazarali and Sarah Muttitt, "Comparison of ring block, dorsal penile nerve block, and topical anesthesia for neonatal circumcision," *JAMA*, 1997; 278(24): 2157–62. This study found that the ring block was more effective than the dorsal penile nerve block.

13. Christopher Kirya and Milton W. Werthmann, "Neonatal circumcision and penile dorsal nerve block—a painless procedure," *The Journal of Pediatrics*, 1978; 92(6): 998–1000; Paul S. Williamson and Marvel L. Williamson, "Physiologic stress reduction by a local anesthetic during newborn circumcision," *Pediatrics*, 1983; 71(1): 36–40; Howard J. Stang, Megan R. Gunnar, Leonard Snellman, Lawrence M. Condon and Roberta Kestenbaum, "Local anesthesia for neonatal circumcision: effects on distress and cortisol response," *JAMA*, 1988; 259(10): 1507–11; David M. Spencer, Kimball A. Miller, Michael O'Quinn, Jacqueline P. Tomsovic, Bradley Anderson, Donna Wong and William E. Williams, "Dorsal penile nerve block in neonatal circumcision: chloroprocaine versus lidocaine," *American Journal of Perinatology*, 1992; 9(3): 214–18; Robert M. Arnett, Stephen Jones and Edgar O. Horger III, "Effectiveness of 1% lidocaine dorsal penile nerve block in infant circumcision," *American Journal of Obstetrics and Gynecology*, 1990; 163(3): 1074–80.

14. Peter Szmuk, Tiberiu Ezri, Herzel Ben Hur, Benjamin Caspi, Lilia Priscu and Virgil Priscu, "Regional anaesthesia for circumcision in adults: a comparative study," *Canadian Journal of Anaesthesia*, 1994; 41: 1181–84.

15. Pedro A. Poma, "Painless neonatal circumcision," *International Journal of Gynaecology and Obstetrics*, 1980; 18: 308–9; Paul S. Williamson and Marvel L. Williamson, "Physiologic stress reduction by a local anesthetic during newborn circumcision," *Pediatrics*, 1983; 71(1): 36–40; Howard J. Stang, Megan R. Gunnar, Leonard Snellman, Lawrence M. Condon and Roberta Kestenbaum, "Local anesthesia for neonatal circumcision: effects on distress and cortisol response," *JAMA*, 1988; 259(10): 1507–11; Leonard W. Snellman and Howard J. Stang, "Prospective evaluation of complications of dorsal penile nerve block for neonatal circumcision," *Pediatrics*, 1995, 95(5): 705–8; Janice Lander, Barbara Brady-Fryer, James B. Metcalfe, Shemin Nazarali and Sarah Muttitt, "Comparison of ring block, dorsal penile nerve block, and topical anesthesia for neonatal circumcision," *JAMA*, 1997; 278(24): 2157–62.

16. C. A. Sara and C. J. Lowry, "A complication of circumcision and dorsal block of the penis," *Anaesthesia and Intensive Care*, 1985; 13(1): 79–82.

17. Christopher Kirya and Milton W. Werthmann, "Neonatal circumcision and penile dorsal nerve block—a painless procedure," *The Journal of Pediatrics*, 1978; 92(6): 998–1000; Paul S. Williamson and Marvel L. Williamson, "Physiologic stress reduction by a local anesthetic during newborn circumcision," *Pediatrics*, 1983; 71(1): 36–40; Howard J. Stang, Megan R. Gunnar, Leonard Snellman, Lawrence M. Condon and Roberta Kestenbaum, "Local anesthesia for neonatal circumcision: effects on distress and cortisol response," *JAMA*, 1988; 259(10): 1507–11.

18. Harold Speert, "Circumcision of the newborn: an appraisal of its present status," *Obstetrics and Gynecology*, 1953; 2(2): 164–71.

19. Hawa Patel, "The problem of routine circumcision," *Canadian Medical Association Journal*, 1966; 95: 576–81, 580.

20. William F. Gee and Julian S. Ansell, "Neonatal circumcision: a ten-year overview: with comparison of the Gomco clamp and Plastibell device," *Pediatrics*, 1976; 58(6): 824–27, 824; Thomas E. Wiswell and Dietrich W. Geschke, "Risks from circumcision during the first month of life compared with those for uncircumcised boys," *Pediatrics*, 1989; 83(6): 1011–15, 1011; R. M. Fredman, "Neonatal circumcision: a general practitioner survey," *Medical Journal of Australia*, 1969; 1: 117–20, 119.

21. Harold Speert, "Circumcision of the newborn: an appraisal of its present status," *Obstetrics and Gynecology*, 1953; 2(2): 164–71, 171.

22. George C. Denniston, "Tyranny of the Victims: An analysis of Circumcision Advocacy," in George C. Denniston, Frederick Mansfield Hodges and Marilyn Fayre Milos (Eds.), *Male and Female Circumcision: Medical Legal and Ethical Considerations in Pediatric Practice*, New York: Kluwer, 1999; 221–40, 223. Not everybody accepts these statistics. A recent paper cites data which puts the incidence of penile cancer in the United States at 0.6 per 100,000 males and that in Denmark at 1 per 100,000. [Edgar J. Schoen, Michael Oehrli, Christopher J. Colby and Geoffrey Machin, "The highly protective effect of newborn circumcision against invasive penile cancer," *Pediatrics*, 2000; 105(3): e36–e39.

23. Cited by Edgar J. Schoen, Michael Oehrli, Christopher J. Colby and Geoffrey Machin, "The highly protective effect of newborn circumcision against invasive penile cancer," *Pediatrics*, 2000; 105(3): e36–e39.

24. Edgar J. Schoen, Michael Oehrli, Chrisopher J. Colby and Geoffrey Machin, "The highly protective effect of newborn circumcision against invasive penile cancer," *Pediatrics*, 2000; 105(3): e36–e39.

25. Archie L. Dean, "Epithelioma of the Penis," *Journal of Urology*, 1935; 33: 252–83.

26. Herman Lenowitz and Albert P. Graham, "Carcinoma of the penis," *Journal of Urology*, 1946; 56: 458–84.

27. G. J. Hardner, T. Bhanalaph, G. P. Murphy, D. J. Albert and R. H. Moore, "Carcinoma of the penis: Analysis of therapy in 100 consecutive patients," *Journal of Urology*, 1972; 108: 428–30.

28. R. Dagher, M. L. Selzer, and J. Lapides, "Carcinoma of the penis and the anti-circumcision crusade," *Journal of Urology*, 1973; 110: 79–80.

29. Christopher Maden, Karen J. Sherman, Anna Marie Beckmann, T. Gregory Hislop, Chong-Ze Teh, Rhoda L. Ashley and Janet R. Dorling, "History of circumcision, medical conditions and sexual activity and risk of penile cancer," *Journal of the National Cancer Institute*, 1993; 85: 19–24.

30. Reza S. Malek, John R. Goellner, Thomas F. Smith, Mark J. Espy and Michael R. Cupp, "Human papillomavirus infection and intraepithelial, in situ, and invasive carcinoma of penis," *Urology*, 1993; 42: 159–70.

31. Edgar J. Schoen, Michael Oehrli, Christopher J. Colby and Geoffrey Machin, "The highly protective effect of newborn circumcision against invasive penile cancer," *Pediatrics*, 2000; 105(3); e36–e39.

32. There is conflicting evidence about whether self-report is a reliable way of determining circumcision status. Some studies [for example Marc Urassa, James Todd, J. Ties Boerma,

Richard Hayes and Raphael Isingo, "Male circumcision and susceptibility to HIV infection among men in Tanzania," *AIDS*, 1997; 11(1): 73–80, 78] suggest that it is not, while others [Susan W. Parker, Andrew J. Stewart, Michael N. Wren, Morris M. Gollow and Judith A. Y. Straton, "Circumcision and sexually transmittable disease," *The Medical Journal of Australia*, 1983; 2: 288–90] suggest that it is.

33. Circumcision beyond infancy has not been as well studied but seems not to confer the same magnitude of benefit.

34. Edgar J. Schoen, "The relationship between circumcision and cancer of the penis," *CA. A Cancer Journal for Physicians*, 1991; 41(5): 306–9, 307; Edgar J. Schoen, "Neonatal circumcision and penile cancer," *British Medical Journal*, 1996; 313: 46; Edgar J. Schoen, Michael Oehrli, Christopher J. Colby and Geoffrey Machin, "The highly protective effect of newborn circumcision against invasive penile cancer," *Pediatrics*, 2000; 105(3): e36–e39, e37.

35. George C. Denniston, "Tyranny of the victims: An analysis of circumcision advocacy," in George C. Denniston, Frederick Mansfield Hodges and Marilyn Fayre Milos (Eds.), *Male and Female Circumcision: Medical Legal and Ethical Considerations in Pediatric Practice*, New York: Kluwer, 1999; 223–24.

36. Opponents of circumcision typically do not distinguish between the different forms of the disease, and when they do, they do not provide primary data to show that the more severe forms occur in equal or greater degrees in those who are neonatally circumcised.

37. C. M. Ginsberg and G. H. McCracken Jr., "Urinary tract infections in young infants," *Pediatrics*, 1982; 69: 409–11; Thomas E. Wiswell, Franklin R. Smith, James W. Bass, "Decreased incidence of urinary tract infections in circumcised male infants," *Pediatrics*, 1985; 75: 901–3; Thomas W. Wiswell and John D. Roscelli, "Corroborative evidence for the decreased incidence of urinary tract infections in circumcised male infants," *Pediatrics*, 1986; 78: 96–99; Thomas E. Wiswell, Robert W. Enzenauer, J. Devn Cornish and Charles T. Hankins, "Declining frequency of circumcision: Implications for changes in the absolute incidence and male to female sex ratio of urinary tract infections in early infancy," *Pediatrics*, 1987; 79: 338–41; Lynn W. Herzog, "Urinary tract infections and circumcision," *American Journal of Diseases of Children*, 1989; 143: 348–50; T. E. Wiswell and Wayne E. Hachey, "Urinary tract infections and the uncircumcised state: An update," *Clincial Pediatrics*, 1993; 32: 130–34; Teresa To, Mohammad Aghar, Paul T. Dick and William Feldman, "Cohort study on circumcision of newborn boys and subsequent risk of urinary tract infection," *Lancet*, 1998; 352: 1813–16.

38. American Academy of Pediatrics Task Force on Circumcision (Edgar J. Schoen, Glen Anderson, Constance Bohon, Frank Hinman Jr., Ronald Poland and E. Maurice Wakeman), "Report of the task force on circumcision," *Pediatrics*, 1989, 84: 399–91, 389; Edgar J. Schoen, "The status of circumcision of newborns," *New England Journal of Medicine*, 1990; 322: 1308–11,1309; Theodore G. Ganiats, Jonathan B. C. Humphrey, Howard L. Taras and Robert M. Kaplan, "Routine neonatal circumcision: A cost-utility analysis," *Medical Decision Making*, 1991; 11: 282–89, 284; Frank H. Lawler, Roberto S. Bisonni and David R. Holtgrave, "Circumcision: A decision analysis of its medical value," *Family Medicine*, 1991; 23: 587–93, 588; S. Daniel Niku, Jeffrey A. Stock and George W. Kaplan, "Neonatal circumcision," *Urologic Clinics of North America*, 1995; 22: 57–65, 59; Stephen Moses, Robert C. Bailey and Allan R. Ronald, "Male circumcision: assessment of health benefits and risks," *Sexually Transmitted Infections*, 1998; 74: 370–71; and Edgar J. Schoen, Thomas E. Wiswell and Stephen Moses, "New policy on circumcision—cause for concern," *Pediatrics*, 2000; 105: 620–23, 620. Even those papers which conclude that, all things considered, the costs and benefits of circumcision cancel out one another, take the prevention of UTI to be a beneficial feature of circumcision. See, for example: Fetus and Newborn Committee, Canadian Paediatric Society, "Neonatal circumcision revisited," *Canadian Medical Association Journal*, 1996; 154: 371–72; American Academy of Pediatrics Task Force on Circumcision (Carole M. Lannon, Ann Geryl Doll Bailey, Alan R. Fleischman, George W. Kaplan, Graig T. Shoemaker, Jack T. Lawson and Donald Coustan), "Circumcision policy statement," *Pediatrics*, 1999; 103: 689–90; and American Academy of Pediatrics, "Circumcision: Information for parents," www.aap.org/family/circ.htm (accessed 2 January 2001).

39. Teresa To, Mohammad Aghar, Paul T. Dick and William Feldman, "Cohort study on circumcision of newborn boys and subsequent risk of urinary tract infection," *Lancet*, 1998; 352: 1813–16.

40. T. E. Wiswell and Wayne E. Hachey, "Urinary tract infections and the uncircumcised state: An update," *Clinical Pediatrics*, 1993; 32: 130–34. This is the conclusion of their meta-analysis of nine published studies. Individual studies estimated the increase from 5- to 89-fold.

41. J. M. Littlewood, "66 infants with urinary tract infection in first month of life," *Archives of Disease in Childhood*, 1972; 47: 218–26. This study points to the occurrence of severe complications but overestimates their frequency because it includes a number of cases that were inadequately treated or not treated with antibiotics at all.

42. R. A. Wilson, "Circumcision and venereal disease," *Canadian Medical Association Journal*, 1947; 56: 54–56; Susan W. Parker, Andrew J. Stewart, Michael N. Wren, Morris M. Gollow and Judith A. Y. Straton, "Circumcision and sexually transmittable disease," *The Medical Journal of Australia*, 1983; 2: 288–90; J. Newell, K. Senkoro, F. Mosha, H. Grosskurth, A. Nicoll, L. Barongo, M, Borgdorff, A Klokke, J. Changalucha, J. Killewo, J. Velema, A. S. Muller, J. Rugemalila, D. Maybe and R. Hayes, "A population-based study of syphilis and sexually transmitted disease syndromes in north-western Tanzania. 2. Risk factors and health seeking behaviour," *Genitourinary Medicine*, 1993; 69: 421–26; Linda S. Cook, Laura A. Koutsky and King K. Holmes, "Circumcision and sexually transmitted diseases," *American Journal of Public Health*, 1994; 84: 197–201.

43. Edward O. Laumann, Christopher M. Masi and Ezra W. Zuckerman, "Circumcision in the United States: Prevalence, prophylactic effects and sexual practice," *JAMA*, 1997; 277(13): 1052–57.

44. J. D. J. Parker and J. E. Banatvala, "Herpes genitalis: Clinical and virological studies," *British Journal of Venereal Disease*, 1967; 43; 212–16; P. K. Taylor and P. Rodin, "Herpes genitalis and circumcision," *British Journal of Venereal Disease*, 1975; 51: 274–77; Susan W. Parker, Andrew J. Stewart, Michael N. Wren, Morris M. Gollow and Judith A. Y. Straton, "Circumcision and sexually transmittable disease," *The Medical Journal of Australia*, 1983; 2: 288–90.

45. Edward O. Laumann, Christopher M. Masi and Ezra W. Zuckerman, "Circumcision in the United States: Prevalence, prophylactic effects and sexual practice," *JAMA*, 1997; 277(13): 1052–57; Linda S. Cook, Laura A. Koutsky and King K. Holmes, "Circumcision and sexually transmitted diseases," *American Journal of Public Health*, 1994; 84: 197–201; B. Donovan, I. Bassett and N. J. Bodsworth, "Male circumcision and common sexually transmissible diseases in a developed nation setting," *Genitourinary Medicine*, 1994; 70: 317–20.

46. J. Neil Simonsen, William Cameron, Michael N. Gakinya, Jackoniah Ndinya-Achola, Lourdes J. D'Costa, Peter Karasira, Mary Cheang, Allan R. Ronald, Peter Piot and Francis A. Plummer, "Human immunodeficiency virus infection among men with sexually transmitted diseases. Experience from a center in Africa," *New England Journal of Medicine* 1988; 319(5): 274–78.

47. D. William Cameron, J. Neil Simonsen, Lourdes J. D'Costa, Allan R. Ronald, Gregory M. Maitha, Michael N. Gakinya, Mary Cheang, J. O. Ndinya-Achola, Peter Piot, Robert C. Brunham and Francis A. Plummer, "Female to male transmission of human immunodeficiency virus type 1: risk factors for seroconversion in men," *Lancet*, 1989; ii: 403–7; James M. Nasio, Nico J. D. Nagelkerke, Anthony Mwatha, Stephen Moses, Jackoniah O. Ndinya-Achola and Frank A. Plummer, "Genital ulcer disease among STD clinic attenders in Nairobi: Association with HIV-1 and circumcision status," *International Journal of STD & AIDS*, 1996; 7: 410–14.

48. R. A. Wilson, "Circumcision and venereal disease," *Canadian Medical Association Journal*, 1947; 56: 54–56; Susan W. Parker, Andrew J. Stewart, Michael N. Wren, Morris M. Gollow and Judith A. Y. Straton, "Circumcision and sexually transmittable disease," *The Medical Journal of Australia*, 1983; 2: 288–90; Linda S. Cook, Laura A. Koutsky and King K. Holmes, "Circumcision and sexually transmitted diseases," *American Journal of Public Health*, 1994; 84: 197–201, 198.

49. P. K. Taylor and P. Rodin, "Herpes genitalis and circumcision," *British Journal of Venereal Disease*, 1975; 51: 274–77; Gregory L. Smith, Robert Greenup and Ernest Takafuji, "Circumcision

as a risk factor for urethritis in racial groups," *American Journal of Public Health*, 1987; 77(4): 452–54; B. Donovan, I. Bassett and N. J. Bodsworth, "Male circumcision and common sexually transmissible diseases in a developed nation setting," *Genitourinary Medicine*, 1994; 70: 317–20; Edward O. Laumann, Christopher M. Masi and Ezra W. Zuckerman, "Circumcision in the United States: Prevalence, prophylactic effects and sexual practice," *JAMA*, 1997; 277(13): 1052–57.

50. Gregory L. Smith, Robert Greenup and Ernest Takafuji, "Circumcision as a risk factor for urethritis in racial groups," *American Journal of Public Health*, 1987; 77(4): 452–54; J. Newell, K. Senkoro, F. Mosha, H. Grosskurth, A. Nicoll, L. Barongo, M, Borgdorff, A Klokke, J. Changalucha, J. Killewo, J. Velema, A. S. Muller, J. Rugemalila, D. Maybe and R. Hayes, "A population-based study of syphilis and sexually transmitted disease syndromes in north-western Tanzania. 2. Risk factors and health seeking behaviour," *Genitourinary Medicine*, 1993; 69: 421–26.

51. Susan W. Parker, Andrew J. Stewart, Michael N. Wren, Morris M. Gollow and Judith A. Y. Straton, "Circumcision and sexually transmittable disease," *The Medical Journal of Australia*, 1983; 2: 288–90; Linda S. Cook, Laura A. Koutsky and King K. Holmes, "Circumcision and sexually transmitted diseases," *American Journal of Public Health*, 1994; 84: 197–201, 198; B. Donovan, I. Bassett and N. J. Bodsworth, "Male circumcision and common sexually transmissible diseases in a developed nation setting," *Genitourinary Medicine*, 1994; 70: 317–20; Edward O. Laumann, Christopher M. Masi and Ezra W. Zuckerman, "Circumcision in the United States: Prevalence, prophylactic effects and sexual practice," *JAMA*, 1997; 277(13): 1052–57.

52. Linda S. Cook, Laura A. Koutsky and King K. Holmes, "Circumcision and sexually transmitted diseases," *American Journal of Public Health*, 1994; 84: 197–201, 198; L. S. Cook, L. A. Koutsky and K. K. Holmes, "Clinical presentation of genital warts among circumcised and uncircumcised heterosexual men attending an urban STD clinic," *Genitourinary Medicine*, 1993; 69: 262–64.

53. Susan W. Parker, Andrew J. Stewart, Michael N. Wren, Morris M. Gollow and Judith A. Y. Straton, "Circumcision and sexually transmittable disease," *The Medical Journal of Australia*, 1983; 2: 288–90; B. Donovan, I. Bassett and N. J. Bodsworth, "Male circumcision and common sexually transmissible diseases in a developed nation setting," *Genitourinary Medicine*, 1994; 70: 317–20.

54. Robert S. Van Howe, "Does circumcision influence sexually transmitted diseases? A literature review," *British Journal of Urology International*, 1999, 83 (supplement 1): 52–62, 59.

55. Ibid.

56. American Academy of Pediatrics Task Force on Circumcision, "Circumcision policy statement," *Pediatrics*, 1999; 103(3): 686–93.

57. Ibid, p. 691.

58. Edgar J. Schoen, Thomas E. Wiswell and Stephen Moses, "New policy on circumcision—cause for concern," *Pediatrics*, 2000; 105(3): 620–23, 621.

59. Stephen Moses, Robert C. Bailey and Allan R. Ronald, "Male circumcision: Assessment of health benefits and risk," *Sexually Transmitted Infections*, 1998; 74: 368–73, 370.

60. We refer here to susceptibility to HIV infection rather than to infectivity.

61. Stephen Moses, Francis Plummer, Janet E. Bradley, Jeckoniah O. Ndinya-Achola, Nico J. D. Nagelkerke and Allan R. Ronald, "The association between lack of male circumcision and risk for HIV infection: A review of the epidemiological data," *Sexually Transmitted Diseases*, 1994; 21(4): 201–10.

62. Helen A. Weiss, Maria A. Quigley and Richard J. Hayes, "Male circumcision and risk of HIV infection in sub-Saharan Africa: A systematic review and meta-analysis," *AIDS*, 2000; 14(15): 2361–70.

63. R. S. Van Howe, "Circumcision and HIV infection: Review of the literature and meta-analysis," *International Journal of STD & AIDS*, 1999; 10: 8–16.

64. Stephen Moses, Nico J. D. Nagelkerke and James Blanchard, "Analysis of the scientific literature on male circumcision and the risk for HIV infection," *International Journal of STD & AIDS*, 1999; 10: 626–28.

65. Nigel O'Farrell and Matthias Egger, "Circumcision in men and the prevention of HIV infection: A 'meta-analysis' revisited," *International Journal of STD & AIDS*, 2000; 11(3): 137–42.

66. Stephen Moses, Francis Plummer, Janet E. Bradley, Jeckoniah O. Ndinya-Achola, Nico J. D. Nagelkerke and Allan R. Ronald, "The association between lack of male circumcision and risk for HIV infection: A review of the epidemiological data," *Sexually Transmitted Diseases*, 1994; 21(4): 201–10.

67. Helen A. Weiss, Maria A. Quigley and Richard J. Hayes, "Male circumcision and risk of HIV infection in sub-Saharan Africa: A systematic review and meta-analysis," *AIDS*, 2000; 14(15): 2361–70, 2362.

68. Mark W. Tyndall, Allan R. Ronald, Elizabeth Agoki, William Malisa, Job J. Bwayo, J. O. Ndinya-Achola, Stephen Moses and Francis A. Plummer, "Increased risk of infection with human immunodeficiency virus type 1 among uncircumcised men presenting with genital ulcer disease in Kenya," *Clinical Infectious Diseases*, 1996; 23; 449–53, 450; James M. Nasio, Nico J. D. Nagelkerke, Anthony Mwatha, Stephen Moses, Jackoniah O. Ndinya-Achola and Frank A. Plummer, "Genital ulcer disease among STD clinic attenders in Nairobi: Association with HIV-1 and circumcision status," *International Journal of STD & AIDS*, 1996; 7: 410–14, 411; Gregory L. Smith, Robert Greenup and Ernest Takafuji, "Circumcision as a risk factor for urethritis in racial groups," *American Journal of Public Health*, 1987; 77(4): 452–54: 452; Susan W. Parker, Andrew J. Stewart, Michael N. Wren, Morris M. Gollow and Judith A. Y. Straton, "Circumcision and sexually transmittable disease," *The Medical Journal of Australia*, 1983; 2: 288–90, 288; Linda S. Cook, Laura A. Koutsky and King K. Holmes, "Circumcision and sexually transmitted diseases," *American Journal of Public Health*, 1994; 84: 197–201, 198.

69. Robert C. Bailey, Stella Neema and Richard Othieno, "Sexual behaviors and other HIV risk factors in circumcised and uncircumcised men in Uganda," *Journal of Acquired Immune Deficiency Syndromes*, 1999; 22(3), 294–301.

70. Helen A. Weiss, Maria A. Quigley and Richard J. Hayes, "Male circumcision and risk of HIV infection in sub-Saharan Africa: A systematic review and meta-analysis," *AIDS*, 2000; 14(15): 2361–70, 2363.

71. Linda S. Cook, Laura A. Koutsky and King K. Holmes, "Circumcision and sexually transmitted diseases," *American Journal of Public Health*, 1994; 84: 197–201, 199.

72. Jakob Oster, "Further fate of the foreskin: Incidence of preputial adhesions, phimosis and smegma among Danish schoolboys," *Archives of Diseases of Children*, 1968; 43: 200–203; Heather Krueger and Lucy Osborn, "Effects of hygiene among the uncircumcised," *The Journal of Family Practice*, 1986; 22(4): 353–55; Lynn W. Herzog and Susanna R. Alvarez, "The frequency of foreskin problems in uncircumcised children," *American Journal of Diseases of Children*, 1986; 140: 254–56; D. M. Fergusson, J. M. Lawton and F. T. Shannon, "Neonatal circumcision and penile problems: An eight year longitudinal study," *Pediatrics*, 1988; 81: 537–41.

73. Acquired inability to retract the foreskin.

74. Inability of the retracted foreskin to return to its resting position covering the glans.

75. See for example, Lynn W. Herzog, Susanna R. Alvarez, "The frequency of foreskin problems in uncircumcised children," *American Journal of Diseases of Children*, 1986; 140: 254–56. Some studies have appropriately cautioned against the overdiagnosis of phimosis, given that it is developmentally normal for the foreskin to be unretractable in young children.

76. Inflammation of the glans.

77. Lynn W. Herzog and Susanna R. Alvarez, "The frequency of foreskin problems in uncircumcised children," *American Journal of Diseases of Children*, 1986; 140: 254–56.

78. Inflammation of the meatus.

79. A. Ranald Mackenzie, "Meatal ulceration following neonatal circumcision," *Obstetrics and Gynecology*, 1966; 28(2): 221–23.

80. S. Daniel Niku, Jeffrey A. Stock and George W. Kaplan, "Neonatal circumcision," *Urologic Clinics of North America*, 1995; 22(1): 57–65, 60; Fetus and Newborn Committee, Canadian Paediatric Society, "Neonatal circumcision revisited," *Canadian Medical Association Journal*, 1996;

154: 371–72; Stephen Moses, Robert C. Bailey, Allan R. Ronald, "Male circumcision: Assessment of health benefits and risks," *Sexually Transmitted Infections*, 1998; 74: 370–71.

81. W. H. Masters and V. E. Johnson, *Human Sexual Response*, Boston, MA: Little Brown & Company, 1966; 189–91.

82. Edward O. Laumann, Christopher M. Masi and Ezra W. Zuckerman, "Circumcision in the United States: Prevalence, prophylactic effects and sexual practice," *JAMA*, 1997; 277(13): 1052–57.

83. Frank H. Lawler, Roberto S. Bisonni and David R. Holtgrave, "Circumcision: A decision analysis of its medical value," *Family Medicine*, 1991; 23(8): 587–93; Theodore G. Ganiats, Jonathan B. C. Humphrey, Howard L. Taras and Robert M. Kaplan, "Routine neonatal circumcision: A cost-utility analysis," *Medical Decision Making*, 1991; 11(4): 282–93.

84. At least this is what our discussions with pediatric urologists and gynecologists with interests in this topic suggest.

85. Moses Maimonides, *The Guide for the Perplexed*, New York: Dover Publications (Second Edition), 1956; 378. (Translated by M. Friedländer.) David Gollaher, *Circumcision*, New York: Basic Books, 2000; 102–4.

86. One example is the defeat of what has been termed the "Seattle Compromise." The Harborview Medical Center in Seattle was faced with repeated requests from immigrant Somalian mothers to have their daughters circumcised. The mothers indicated that their daughters would be circumcised with or without the doctors. The hospital suggested a compromise procedure whereby the clitoral prepuce would merely be nicked to draw blood. Evidently this would have satisfied at least some of the mothers. However, even though no tissue would have been removed in this proposed procedure, the plan was squashed by those who oppose any nontherapeutic procedure on a girl's genitalia. Those children who would have had the compromise procedure but who were instead subjected to the traditional one were clearly less well off than they would otherwise have been. [Doriane Lambelet Coleman, "The Seattle compromise: Multicultural sensitivity and Americanization," *Duke Law Journal*, 1998: 47: 717–83.]

87. The use of the term *surgery* is not intended to exclude what are ostensibly surgical procedures but which are performed by non-doctors (such as ritual circumcisers).

88. The distinction between medical and nonmedical benefits is not as sharp as many people may think, but we ignore this problem here.

# 2

## ✝

# The Ethics of Neonatal Male Circumcision: Helping Parents to Decide

## *Leslie Cannold*

The ethics of male circumcision has received little attention in the bioethical literature. In one of the few considerations of the subject, Michael and David Benatar (2003) investigate whether the practice can be justified by examining whether circumcision constitutes bodily mutilation, whether the absence of the child's informed consent makes it wrong, the nature and strength of the evidence regarding medical harms and benefits, and what moral weight cultural considerations have. The Benatars argue that a moral assessment of neonatal circumcision cannot be made without considering its medical costs and benefits. Having provided a thorough assessment on these grounds,[1] they conclude, on the basis of the evenly weighted evidence for and against the procedure, that it is a discretionary medical matter best left to parents to decide on the basis of their own values.

I agree with the Benatars' conclusion that neonatal circumcision is a decision rightly left in the hands of parents. To demonstrate that it is not, it would be necessary to show that the procedure was mutilation or otherwise threatened the health and safety of a child to a degree necessary to justify a societal override of what both legal and ethical precedents have long held to be both a parent's right and responsibility: to make judgments based on their own values about what is in their child's best interests. The Benatars argue persuasively that neither charge, at least on current evidence, can be sustained.[2]

However, claiming that parents should retain the authority to make decisions for their infant boys about circumcision says little about how parents charged with such a decision ought to make it. Circumcision is an invasive medical procedure, and one function of informed consent is to ensure that patients are protected from harm with regard to such procedures. Because

infants cannot themselves consent to circumcision or other medical procedures, parents are charged with giving such consent on their behalf. Ensuring that consent is informed facilitates the fulfillment of their obligation to
protect their child's best interests. These interests include the child's present
and future physical and psychological health and well-being as well as his
stake in becoming an autonomous agent in the future capable of making
medical and other important life choices for himself.

In this chapter, I will discuss the range of issues—medical, ethical, social,
and religious/cultural—that I believe parents must canvass and weigh up in
order to give informed consent to circumcising their neonate.

## INFORMED CONSENT AND PROXY DECISION MAKING

The notion of "informed consent" arose to describe decision-making procedures necessary to protect patients and research participants from harm.
The U.S. Tuskegee syphilis study and the New Zealand "Unfortunate"
cervical cancer experiment are only the most well-known examples of
where failure to inform patients about the nature and risks/benefits of
medical research or therapy caused serious patient harm. More recently,
informed consent has become primarily understood as a means of protecting patient autonomy. If a patient autonomously authorizes her medical practitioner to undertake a particular intervention, then she has given
her informed consent. The two important characteristics of a consent that
is informed are that it is intentionally given by a patient with "substantial
understanding and in substantial absence of control by others"
(Beauchamp and Childress 1994, 143).

A proxy decision maker is required when a person lacks, either temporarily or permanently, the competence to consent for herself. In the case of
neonates, parents are seen to be the most suitable people to act as proxies
because—unless shown otherwise—they are assumed to have their child's
best interests at heart. However, because neonates have never been autonomous, parents cannot make the circumcision decision on the basis of
what they believe their son *would* want were he competent—a standard of
decision making known as *substituted judgment*. Instead, Beauchamp and
Childress (1994) argue that parents must make their decisions on the basis of
what is in their child's best interests, as assessed by their evaluation of what
benefits and burdens the intervention is likely to cause.

The informed consent requirement mitigates the child-patient's risk by ob-
ligating medical professionals to ensure parent-proxies have a substantial
understanding of the risks and benefits of the procedure and have freely
consented to it. At the same time, it provides parents with a clear standard
against which their discharge of their duties as proxy medical decision makers can be measured. Indeed, Ford (2001) argues that unless parents' consent

for their children to have (nonemergency) medical interventions is fully informed, their decisions lack not just ethical but also legal standing.

So what specific issues must a parent gain a substantial understanding of, and give weight to, in order to make an informed decision about circumcising their neonate? In my view, these include considerations of a medical, ethical, social, and religious/cultural nature.

## NEONATAL CIRCUMCISION:
## PARENTAL MOTIVES, PARENTAL CONSIDERATIONS

Parents have different reasons for considering circumcision for their neonate. For some parents, the question of whether or not to circumcise is a medical one, while for others social concerns (e.g., ensuring their son will look like his dad) are predominant. Historically, circumcision was a religious and cultural ritual, and both the Jewish and Muslim traditions continue to demand parents circumcise their children when young.[3]

These different motives mean that not all parents will or should need to consider all the matters that may be of relevance to the decisions of some. To take the most obvious example, while the religious or cultural beliefs or affiliations may be central to Jewish and Muslim parents, such beliefs and affiliations will not and need not feature in the considerations of parents with no such religious or cultural beliefs or ties. However, some aspects of the circumcision decision should feature in the consideration of all parents. Usually, these have included tangible factors like physical and financial risks, harms, and benefits (Beauchamp and Childress 1989, 171), but can—and insofar as circumcision is concerned, I would argue, should—take in social, psychological, and spiritual risks, benefits, and burdens of the procedure. This means that while requirements for informed consent vary among parents, there exists a minimum suite of considerations which all parents should consider relevant to their child's best interests. Parents must canvass such considerations for them to satisfy their responsibility to make an informed and voluntary decision about neonatal circumcision.

### Medical

The position of leading medical organizations in the United States, Canada, New Zealand, and Australia (among others) is that there is no medical indication for routine neonatal circumcision (Circinfo.org 2003; CIRP 2004). Moreover, the review of the medical evidence provided by the Benatars shows that the costs and benefits of circumcision are more or less evenly balanced. How should parents respond to these conclusions, which can be summed up as "there are no medical reasons for or against circumcision"?

Declines in the neonatal circumcision rate in many countries following the medical community's rejection of it as a routine procedure suggest that for many parents such authoritative conclusions about the procedure's lack of *net* medical value will be decisive.[4] However, this will not be the case for all parents. This is because, in keeping with their obligation to make the decision based on their assessment of their own child's best interests, some parents will find, among the costs and benefits of circumcision, something they deem particularly relevant to the decision they make about their child. For instance, parents of a premature baby forced to endure numerous painful medical interventions in the early weeks of his life may see the primary interest of their child as being the avoidance of further unnecessary pain,[5] and reject neonatal circumcision on this basis. Alternatively, a father with a long history of painful urinary tract infections (UTIs) may be extremely concerned to see his son avoid this burden as in infant. Having noted that existing medical evidence shows circumcision can protect against childhood UTIs, he may deem the procedure to be in his child's best interests.[6]

## Ethical

Beauchamp and Childress (1994) argue that unless parents can answer the question "What would the patient want in this circumstance?" they are unable to make decisions for their infant according to the "substituted judgment" standard, or in the way they would for their baby son if he had once been competent. It is because the newborn has never been competent, and therefore that there is no basis for a judgment of autonomous choice, that parents must decide for their infants on the basis of their own assessment of their child's best interests.

However, their newborn's current incompetency does not mean that parental concerns about their child's autonomy and privacy should disappear from their considerations about circumcision. This is because most newborns will one day acquire the competency necessary to make autonomous decisions about circumcision and other medical and life issues. Indeed, as Ross has argued, one of the obligations parents have is to "promote their child's growth and development" so they can become such independent autonomous agents (1993, 1).

Anticircumcision literature abounds with anecdotal evidence that some adult men who are unhappy about being circumcised feel angry about the fact that their parents' decision about the circumcision deprived them of the capacity to make their own autonomous choice about the procedure.[7] The quality of data on this question is low.[8] However, there seems enough evidence to suggest that an indeterminate number of men will express dissatisfaction with their circumcised status, and that among these will be men angry about being compelled to live with the consequences of a decision they had no input into or control over and which they cannot alter, at least not easily or well.[9]

To answer the charge that parents have no right to make the circumcision decision for their neonate (whether the charge is made by a disgruntled adult son circumcised as a neonate or by organized opponents of neonatal circumcision) requires consideration of the validity of reasons parents have for believing that the decision about circumcision must be made when the child is an infant, and therefore by them on their child's behalf. Certainly there are nonemergency medical decisions that parents are justified—on the grounds of the child's best interests—in making before the child is old enough to give his own consent. The question is, is circumcision one of them?

Before answering this question, it is necessary to discuss the question of child competency. Competency, which Beauchamp and Childress define as "the ability to perform a task," is not an all-or-nothing affair in either children or adults. Instead it makes sense to talk about a person's competency to undertake a particular task: in this case, consenting to circumcision. When might a boy obtain the competence to make the circumcision decision himself? The courts, political decision makers, and society at large have devoted attention to the question of when children are competent to decide about weighty medical matters,[10] because of the challenge antichoice activists consistently pose to the validity of the decisions young women make about abortion.[11] In the landmark English *Gillick* case, the judge ruled that children under 16 should be deemed competent to consent to medical treatment when they are capable of making a reasonable assessment of the advantages and disadvantages of the treatment proposed (Devereux 1991). Beauchamp and Childress state the requirements for competence in more detail, but contend similarly that if the child can understand information material to their decision, make a judgment about it in light of his values, intend a certain outcome, and freely communicate his wishes to his doctor, then he is autonomous enough to make the decision by and for himself. While there is not a great deal of evidence available about the validity of children's consent to medical treatment, one survey found that the capacity of most 14-year-olds to give informed consent was indistinguishable from that of adults (Devereux 1991, 300). Thus, it is likely that, somewhere around the age of 14, boys will be competent to decide for themselves about circumcision.

It seems valid for parents to choose circumcision for their neonate when the benefits of the procedure they hope to gain for their child—and which they believe are in his best interest—will be reaped partially or in total prior to the child becoming competent to make the decision himself. Circumcising to protect their infant and young child from UTIs is a good example of this sort of choice. However, the same cannot be said if the claimed medical advantage parents find compelling is likely to be reaped by their child *after* he becomes competent to decide about circumcision himself. The reduction in

risk of human immunodeficiency virus (HIV) transmission is a good example of this sort of advantage. If there are no compelling reasons why—in order to serve the child's best interests—parents need to circumcise before the
child attains competence, then parents should choose to foster their child's
future autonomy by refraining from making the circumcision decision for
him. Instead, they should wait until he has attained the capacity to decide
for himself, and by so doing preserve what Feinberg (1980) calls the child's
right to an "open future."[12]

## Social

There are two commonly cited social reasons that parents seek circumcision:
the belief that the circumcised penis is easier to keep clean,[13] and a desire for
the child to "look like dad" or other male family members.[14]

### Hygiene

There is no evidence that the uncircumcised penis poses significantly more
difficulties either for parents or, as a boy grows, the child himself, to keep
clean. Indeed, in the early years, retraction of the foreskin is contraindicated,
making the hygiene requirements of uncircumcised boys identical to those
without foreskins. Only as the child grows and can, by himself and with
ease, retract the foreskin does this need to be done on a daily basis for cleaning. For most boys, retraction will become possible somewhere between the
ages of 5 and 10. The question is, once retractable, are the cleaning requirements of the uncircumcised penis onerous and, if so, does this justify a parents' decision to circumcise?

   The claim that the hygiene demands of intact children are more onerous than
circumcised ones is highly contestable. Most children have a nightly bath or
shower and, when retraction becomes possible, the cleaning process is approximately a 5- to 10-second operation. Given this, it is hard to imagine how either
the performing of this task by the parent, or the job parents have to remind the
child to do it, could be called onerous (or any more onerous than cleaning, or
reminding them to clean, behind their ears!). Thus it seems to me that the belief that hygiene requirements of an uncircumcised boy are more onerous than
those of a circumcised child is a false one—and making a decision to circumcise on the basis of it is inadequately informed. Moreover, the solution of circumcision to the parental problem of hygiene may fall foul of demands for consistency. As one 5-year-old American boy noted in response to his mother's
explanation that some parents circumcised their sons because they worried that
if they didn't, their boys wouldn't keep clean: "Well, that's dumb, Mom!! What
are they gonna do? Cut their butts off, too?!"[15]

   In addition, parents who choose circumcision to relieve themselves of the
burden of caring for a child with an uncircumcised penis may be acting

against their obligation to make the circumcision decision on the basis of their assessment of their child's best interests rather than their own. In instances where there are significant differences in the requirements of caring for a particular child who has or does not have a particular intervention (with one way of proceeding offering outcomes that are significantly less burdensome for parents than others), parents may be able to mount a credible case for or against that intervention on the grounds that their well-being and the child's are interdependent, and therefore what is good for them or the family unit as a whole is, for that reason, also good for the child.[16] However, given the facts about the hygiene requirements of children with foreskins, the circumcision decision clearly doesn't qualify.

*Just Like Dad*

Logically, there seems no reason for a boy to consider any difference between his penis and that of his dad or other male family members as any more remarkable or significant that any of the myriad of other physical dissimilarities between himself and these others. Further, there seems no evidence that children younger than three notice genitals at all, nor that those older than this take any notice of their or other men's foreskins or—if they do—attribute significance to these differences.[17] My husband is circumcised, but his brother—only four years younger—is not, due to changes in standard Australian hospital practice around the time of their births. Neither man recalls any issue arising over the difference in the look of their members or over the difference between my husband's brother's intact penis and that of their father, who was circumcised. Anecdotal evidence suggests that many adult men are not even sure whether their fathers are or were circumcised. Where children do notice, the meaning they make of the differences they observe seem highly variable. One father tells how his boy was 3 before concluding—his foreskin having retracted of its own accord—that he was "just like Daddy." Daddy, however, was circumcised. The boy is now close to 5, but according to his father is still unaware that he is "different from Daddy" (Ray 1997).

What this suggests is that it may be Dad's or other male relatives' awareness of and anxiety about the difference that motivate parental decisions to circumcise, rather than anticipation of and worry about the child's anxiety on this question. While again, the interactive nature of parent–child relations makes it possible that an anxious father could transmit this anxiety to his son, circumcising in order to rule out this possibility seems a clear case of treating the wrong patient. It would be better to attempt to educate fathers to see the differences in penile appearance between themselves and their sons as just one of the many that do and will continue to mark both their appearances and characters. For in the same way that decisions to circumcise made to ease the perceived hygiene burden of boys with foreskins violate parental obligations to make such choices to foster their sons' best interests, so too do decisions made to ease parental anxieties about bodily differences.

## Cultural/Religious

A number of religions require circumcision. In Islam there seems to be general agreement that circumcision, while encouraged and widely practiced, is not essential, though in Judaism, circumcision is deemed an essential mark for all males. Those who refuse to mark their children thus or, if they are converts, to be circumcised themselves, will—according to the Torah—be "cut off from their kin."[18] While Jews are increasingly questioning the practice of circumcision, it is fair to say that those who believe there is scriptural justification for not undertaking it and are refusing to do so remain in the minority.[19] Thus, for Jewish parents who believe in the importance of following the biblical injunction to ritually circumcise their son and who want their son to be accepted as a member of the Jewish community, circumcision is—in most instances—required.

What does this mean for Jewish parents seeking to make a decision about circumcision for their son? For devout Jews, a failure to circumcise their infant son would clearly be seen as a dereliction of their duty to foster their child's best interests by ensuring he enters properly—meaning through circumcision on the eighth day of his life—into the covenant with God. However, even for Jews who see the requirement to circumcise neonatally as fatally inconsistent with their other values,[20] or even unjustified on theological grounds, the best-interest requirement can mean they feel compelled to circumcise anyway. This is because refusing to circumcise their child may lead the Jewish community to which they belong, and the wider Jewish community, to withhold recognition and acceptance of their child as a Jew, to view them as negligent for refusing to circumcise and, consequently, to exclude or marginalize them all.[21] Parents who see Jewish religious beliefs or identity as their child's birthright or valued gift, and themselves as morally obliged to provide such a gift, would be hard-pressed not to see neonatal circumcision to be in their child's best interests.

## OBJECTIONS

I have argued that while parents are entitled to make the decision to circumcise their male neonate, they are not without responsibilities in the way they go about making this choice. As proxy decision makers, parents are obliged to give informed consent to the procedure being undertaken and, through doing so, ensure that they only authorize the procedure if it can clearly be shown to be in their particular child's best interests.

## Female Genital Mutilation

What does this account suggest about how parents should approach the issue of female genital mutilation (FGM)? Specifically, if the conclusion that parents' religious or cultural beliefs, or parental desires to retain membership in a religious or cultural community, justify male circumcision, doesn't consistency require that parental authorization of FGM be similarly respected?

The simple answer is no. The entitlement parents have to decide about male circumcision is accorded because the procedure is not one that threatens the child's health or well-being. The same cannot be said of FGM, in which anything from part of the clitoris to the entire external female genital organs are excised, leading to—at a minimum—pain for a woman during urination, sex, and/or childbirth, and in a worst-case scenario, the need for surgical intervention in order for a woman to have sex and to give birth. As well, women who have been victims of traditional FGM are at higher risks of pelvic infections, hemorrhaging, obstructed child labor, HIV infection, and even death (Devine et al. 1999). Comparing traditional forms of FGM to male circumcision, according to one commentator, is like equating ear piercing to penectomy (Coleman 1998, 736).

However, the Benatars (2003) argue that the excision of the clitoral prepuce is "anatomically neither more nor less radical a procedure than removal of the penile foreskin," though they do note that while there is some evidence about the medical value of male circumcision, there is none, at least thus far, about the benefits of removing female preputial tissue. *If* it is true that the excision of the clitoral prepuce is analogous to the removal of the penile foreskin, then they are right to suggest that, should evidence of medical benefits for this procedure be discovered, consistency would require that in instances where cultural reasons suffice for undertaking the latter, they should also justify the former. Certainly, I would agree with them that where cultural reasons justify neonatal male circumcision, they would also justify the sort of clitoral "nicking" procedure proposed in the Seattle compromise.[22]

## One Parent or Two? How Many Parents Constitute Consent?

I have argued that the only justification for state interference in parents' medical decisions about their children is when those decisions can clearly be shown to threaten the child's health or safety. But what of instances where parents disagree about whether a particular intervention is in their child's best interests? Specifically, when parents disagree about circumcision, is it justified for the state to intervene and, if so, to what end?

Recently, some anticircumcision activists have begun lobbying for legislation requiring doctors to obtain consent from *both* a child's parents before circumcising their neonate. In Australia, the call for two-parent consent followed a case where an Egyptian father circumcised his two children, ages 5 and 9, against their Australian Aboriginal mother's wishes. The police prosecuted the man for assault, but newspaper reports often failed to reveal that the charges were not grounded in his pursuit of circumcision without his wife's consent, but because a Family Court order existed that specifically prohibited the boy's father from harming them during contact visits.[23] It is hard to escape the feeling that those pursuing such legal change are doing so in order to increase the difficulty parents face in circumcising their child, rather than to protect the best interests of children. While anticircumcision activists would, of course, argue that making it harder for parents to choose circumcision is in the best interests of all male children, acting to whittle away the freedom of parents to make their own informed decisions on the matter is contrary to the ethical and legal requirements of the circumcision decision, which are that parents have the right and responsibility to choose for their own child on the basis of what they believe to be in their particular child's best interests.

However, when parents fail to resolve disagreements about matters of critical importance to the child's health and welfare—and here I would include circumcision—they invite state interference (typically in the form of the Family Court) to examine the evidence and make a ruling. The idea that is at work here, affirmed in numerous U.S. court decisions over the years, is that there is a subjective element to the determination of what constitutes a child's best interests. Indeed, it is this subjective element that has led the courts to leave decisions in which the child's health and safety are not at issue to the parents for them to make according to their own values. But where parents cannot agree about serious matters, there is no alternative—and courts should not hesitate—to step in and produce a "trumping" third-party judgment about what is "best."[24]

In one such case, the objection of a secular English mother to the circumcision of her five-year-old son by his religious father was upheld on the basis that she was primarily raising the boy and doing so in a secular fashion, thereby making circumcision against his best interests. The father appealed the case, but lost.[25] However, the court noted that while circumcision was among a "small group" of "important decisions" that requires the consent of both parents, disagreement between parents about such matters would be settled by the courts on the basis of judgments on the individual facts of a case about what constituted a particular child's best interests.[26] Such rulings in other words, do not and should not be understood to be passing blanket judgments on circumcision, but rather to be applying the best-interest test in the absence of an agreement between parents about how to do so. Such an approach suggests that the state has the same responsibility as parents to ensure they gain a substantial understanding of the issues involved in order that it can make an informed and voluntary decision about whether the procedure will serve the particular child's best interests.

## CONCLUSION

While parents are legally and ethically responsible for decisions regarding neonatal circumcision, this does not mean they lack responsibilities in regard to their decision. Parents are required to make decisions about the procedure in a substantially informed and voluntary manner, and at a minimum to consider the medical and ethical implications of the procedure for their child. An examination of the full range of motives for parental decisions to circumcise reveals that only some medical and religious or cultural ones seem to meet the requirement that such decisions be made to further the best interest of the child, are not based on false beliefs, and fulfill the ethical requirement that parents assume the decision for their incompetent child only when the benefits they see to be in their child's best interests are to be reaped prior to the child becoming competent to make the decision himself.

## NOTES

I am indebted to Neil Levy and Stephen Clarke for helpful comments on earlier drafts.

1. The Benatars consider the issues of neonatal operative and postoperative pain; surgical complications of the procedure; and the relative risks of penile cancer, urinary tract infections, STDs, HIV, phimosis, and paraphimosis in circumcised and uncircumcised boys. They also look at the evidence for claims that genital hygiene is increased in circumcised men relative to those who have not been circumcised, as are the chances of female partners avoiding cervical cancer.

2. One possible counter to this conclusion would be if it could be conclusively demonstrated that circumcision consistently and significantly reduced male sexual pleasure. In this instance, an argument may be able to be made that the procedure does seriously threaten a child's health and safety and so does constitute an unjustified assault on their person. However, as the Benatars rightly note, there is little objective information about the impact of circumcision on male sexuality, and what does exist is contradictory (with some studies saying circumcision has no impact on male sexual pleasure, others concluding it does, while still others report less sexual dysfunction in circumcised males and a preference for circumcised men among female partners (Laumann, Masi et al. 1997; Masters and Johnson 1966). As a consequence of this uncertainty, I have left the matter of sexual pleasure to one side of this discussion.

3. The Jewish prescription is for ritual circumcision eight days after the child's birth unless the child is unhealthy, in which case the procedure is prohibited. The Islamist tradition is more flexible. While the preferred time is the seventh day after birth, circumcision can be carried out up to 40 days after the child is born or thereafter until the age of 7 years, depending upon the child's health and circumstances (Islam Online 2004).

4. Patel (1966) argues that where medical practitioners oppose the procedure, approximately 20 percent of neonate boys will be circumcised at the insistence of their parents. It is possible, however, that such figures will vary on a country-by-country basis, with rates likely to be higher, regardless of medical attitudes, in countries with long cultural/religious histories of the practice and lower in those without.

5. Few dispute the ability of newborns to experience pain, or that circumcision—the actual procedure and its aftermath—causes it. While interventions deemed to be effective in relieving the pain of circumcision and the aftermath are available, they are not always used, as disagreement exists about ease of administration, risks involved in use in newborns, and

the amount of pain caused by the interventions themselves (Benatar and Benatar 2003, 36–37).

6. The Benatars' (2003) review of the evidence led them to suggest circumcision provides a "small but real" benefit of lowering the incidence of UTIs.

7. Circumcision Information Australia notes that they have "received many complaints from adult men who are unhappy about having been circumcised as infants or children. . . . Only the owner of the penis has the right to decide if he would like its appearance, structure and function altered by circumcision or any other needless procedure." Or as one man on the British anticircumcision website Norm.UK.org put it, "I've never expressed my outrage to anyone before, but I do know that the realisation in my late teens that I had had a very important bit of me removed unnecessarily at someone's whim, had a profound effect on me."

8. The one study of psychological consequences reported in the literature was done by Hammond (1999). Among the 546 men he surveyed, he found circumcised men reported "emotional distress, manifesting as intrusive thoughts about one's circumcision, included feelings of mutilation (60%), low self-esteem/inferiority to intact men (50%), genital dysmorphia (55%), rage (52%), resentment/depression (59%), violation (46%), or parental betrayal (30%)." However, the recruitment method of the survey, from among men who had contacted anticircumcision organizations, raises serious questions about the applicability of the findings to the general population of circumcised men.

9. There are men who attempt to reconstruct their foreskin using both surgical and nonsurgical methods. For surgical methods, see Greer, Mohl et al. 1982; Penn 1963; and Goodwin 1990. For nonsurgical, see Bigelow 1995.

10. By age 3 or so, most children are competent to make minor medical decisions like whether or not they want a bandage for a skinned knee. The medical decisions we are discussing here are on the other end of the weightiness scale and therefore require a higher level of competence.

11. My claim here is not that antichoice activists pursue these issues in the court because of sincere concern about the competence of young women to consent to abortion: parental notification/consent laws are a well-established prong of antichoice strategy designed to reduce the incidence of abortion through the creation of all possible legal, bureaucratic, and practical obstacles to women obtaining the procedure "on the ground." All I am arguing here is that when these laws have been challenged, one of the main issues the courts have examined is the competence of the young woman to consent to her own medical treatment: a competence that—if universal—would render such "squeal" laws an unjustified invasion of the woman's entitlement to privacy and/or autonomy. See Puzella 1997 on U.S. law and Devereux 1991 for the situation in the United Kingdom and Australia.

12. One counter to this argument is the contention that neonatal circumcision is a less risky/painful procedure than circumcision done on an older child or adult. However, it seems to me that unless conclusive evidence that this was the case could be presented, which my reading of the current literature suggests it cannot, this argument must fail. Another objection, suggested by Parfit's (1984) example of a man about to undergo painful surgery, might be that even if the pain of circumcision in adulthood is *less* than that experienced by an infant, parents may feel it better to get this pain over with in infancy when the child won't remember it, rather than leave it in the future as pain *to be* experienced and remembered. However, the comparison between past/future benefits (including the experience of pain and memory of that experience) is false because it presumes what is at issue: whether the child, once an adult, will choose circumcision. While it certainly could be the case that an uncircumcised child who decides when he becomes competent that he wants circumcision might resent his parent's failure to have made the choice for him when he was a child because his pain would have been in the past and he would be unable to recollect it, the uncircumcised child who does not wish to be circumcised would not appreciate his parent's decision because even though his pain is in the past and he doesn't recall it, he has been left with the unwanted outcome of their decision: circumcision.

13. Hygiene has both health and social dimensions. Failing to bathe, for instance, may leave you more open to infection, but also makes you smell unpleasant to others. After some consid-

eration, I have decided to describe hygiene as a social consideration because the medical literature does not describe smegma, the creamy yellow sebaceous material that is secreted by the glans and often accumulates in clumps under the foreskin, as a medical problem nor suggest that it indirectly causes any medical problems, little less those that would indicate circumcision. See Simpson 1998.

14. See, for example, Dickey 2002.

15. From http://www.mothersagainstcirc.org/easy.htm.

16. Such discussions arise in discussions of the legitimacy of parents allowing their minor children to become organ donors for relatives. Some experts contend that parents should be allowed to make such proxy decisions about organ donation for their incompetent child grounded not only in the donor child's best interests, but to further the best interests of the family as a whole. See Morley 2002.

17. Freud theorized that somewhere between the ages of 3 and 6, boys become enamored with their mothers and fear castration by their fathers for this love interest and their newfound interest in masturbation. However, Freud's claim is that what boys notice at this age is the difference between their own genitals and those of girls (whom they see as castrated), not differences between their foreskin status and those of other men. Thus, leaving aside the question of the validity of Freudian theory on this point, it is not relevant to the claims I am making here.

18. The relevant passage, from Genesis 17, reads as follows: "As for you, you and your offspring to come throughout the ages shall keep my covenant. Such shall be the covenant between me and you and your offspring to follow, which you shall keep: Every male among you shall be circumcised. You shall circumcise the flesh of your foreskin and that shall be the sign of the covenant between me and you. And throughout the generations every male among you shall be circumcised at the age of eight days. . . . Thus shall my covenant be marked in your flesh as an everlasting pact. And if any male who is uncircumcised fails to circumcise the flesh of his foreskin, that person shall be cut off from his kin. He has broken my covenant."

19. For the religious justifications for not circumcising, see Goldman 1998 and Moss 1991. However, while there is no doubt that a growing number of Jews are rejecting the practice, even Goldman acknowledges that Jewish parents who don't circumcise are in the minority (see Clemente 1998).

20. Jewish parents with feminist beliefs, for instance, can find the practice offensive or unnecessary, given the lack of a similar ceremony by which girls are welcomed into the Jewish community and a sanctified relationship with God. Indeed, in some Jewish communities, alternate nonsurgical ceremonial practices are being developed to serve these purposes for both boy and girl babies (see, for example, Karsenty 1988).

21. I note here that an uncircumcised Jew is still considered a Jew and therefore I am speaking of a social withholding of recognition and acceptance rather than a legal one.

22. The "Seattle compromise" was a procedure developed by a medical center attempting to manage requests from immigrant Somalian mothers to have their daughters circumcised. The procedure, which would have appeased some mothers, was designed to draw blood but not cause any lasting damage to the child's genitals. See Coleman 1998.

There is one important disanalogy between FGM and male circumcision, which is that while FGM is a cultural practice intended to inhibit and/or control the female body and female sexuality, male circumcision is intended as a ritual of inclusion designed to welcome men—and only men—into a special relationship with God. Coleman (1998), a supporter of the Seattle compromise, sees the patriarchal underpinnings of the practice—its essential aim to ensure the physical and cultural domination of women as the reason why Americanization of the immigrants who practice it will and should lead to it withering away in a few generations (the compromise representing a "transitional" measure). However, I am unable to see how the patriarchal nature of FGM as against circumcision provides grounds for altering my conclusions about the range and limits of parental freedom to choose FGM, clitoral nicking, or male circumcision for their children.

23. For an account of the case by an anticircumcision group, and several newspaper articles in which it was reported, see CIRP 2004.

24. U.S. courts have gone even further than this. In *Bellotti* v. *Baird*, the Supreme Court accorded itself the right to authorize a young woman's abortion, even in cases where one or both parents have refused consent and the woman is deemed incompetent to consent herself, when it believes the procedure is in her best interests. The implied view of such judgments seems to be that in the absence of agreement between parents or between a parent and (older) child about what is in the child's best interests, the courts must and will decide. See Lurvey 1990 and Puzella 1997.

25. Re J (child's religious upbringing and circumcision). Jane Maynard Barrister, Family Court. 1 FCR 307 [2000].

26. One of the judges, Dame Elizabeth Butler-Sloss P., argued that a small group of important decisions included sterilization and the change of a child's surname.

# REFERENCES

Beauchamp, T. L., and J. F. Childress. 1989. *Principles of biomedical ethics.* 3rd ed. New York: Oxford University Press.
———. 1994. *Principles of biomedical ethics.* 4th ed. New York: Oxford University Press.
Benatar, M., and D. Benatar. 2003. Between prophylaxis and child abuse: The ethics of neonatal male circumcision. *American Journal of Bioethics* 3 (2): 35–48.
Bigelow, J. 1995. *The joy of uncircumcising! Exploring circumcision; History, myths, psychology, restoration, sexual pleasure and human rights.* 2nd ed. Aptos, CA: Hourglass.
Circinfo.org. 2003. Case study: Forced circumcision in Queensland; Middle Eastern father subjects Australian boys to Islamic rite. *Circumcision Information Australia,* "Legal and Ethical Issues," http://www.circinfo.org/ethics.html.
CIRP. 2004. Circumcision: Medical organization official policy statements. December 3. *Circumcision Information and Resource Pages,* http://www.cirp.org/library/statements.
Clemente, A. L. "Circumcision no longer automatic in Jewish households." *Grand Rapids Press,* May 2, 1998.
Coleman, D. L. 1998. The Seattle compromise: Multicultural sensitivity and Americanization. *Duke Law Journal* 47: 717–83.
Devereux, J. 1991. The capacity of a child in Australia to consent to medical treatment: *Gillick* revisited? *Oxford Journal of Legal Studies* 11 (2): 283–302.
Devine, C., C. R. Hansen, R. Wilde et al. 1999. Female genital mutilation. In *Human rights: The essential reference,* ed. Hilary Poole. Phoenix: Oryx Press.
Dickey, N. 2002. To circumcise or not to circumcise . . . Many parents are asking the question. *Medem,* http://www.medem.com/msphs/msphs_drdickeycolumns_detail.cfm?article_ID=ZZZGMO72B6D.
Feinberg, J. 1980. The right to an open future. In *Whose child? Children's rights, parental authority, and state power,* ed. W. Aiken and H. LaFollette, Totowa, NJ: Rowman and Littlefield. 124–53.
Ford, K.-K. 2001. "First, do no harm": The fiction of legal parental consent to genital-normalizing surgery on intersexed infants. *Yale Law & Policy Review* 19: 469–88.
Goldman, R. 1998. *Questioning circumcision: A Jewish perspective.* Boston: Vanguard.
Goodwin, W. 1990. Uncircumcision: A technique for plastic reconstruction of a prepuce after circumcision. *Journal of Urology* 144: 1203–05.
Greer, D. M., Jr., P. C. Mohl et al. 1982. A technique for foreskin reconstruction and some preliminary results. *Journal of Sex Research* 18 (4): 324–30.
Hammond, T. 1999. A preliminary poll of men circumcised in infancy or childhood. *British Journal of Urology International* 83, suppl. 1: 85–92.
Islam Online. 2004. Medical ethics of male circumcision. February 13. http://www.islamonline.com/cgi-bin/news_service/fatwah_story.asp?service_id=196.
Karsenty, N. 1988. A mother questions *brit milla. Humanistic Judaism* 16 (3): 14–21.

Laumann, E., C. Masi et al. 1997. Circumcision in the United States: Prevalence, prophylactic effects, and sexual practice. *Journal of the American Medical Association* 277 (13): 1052–57.

Lurvey, I. 1990. How many parents constitute parental consent? *Family Advocate* (Fall): 52–53.

Masters, W. H., and V. E. Johnson. 1966. *Human sexual response*. Boston: Little, Brown.

Morley, M. 2002. Proxy consent to organ donation by incompetents. *Yale Law Journal* 111 (5): 1215–49.

Moss, L. B. 1991. The Jewish roots of anti-circumcision arguments. Presentation at the Second International Symposium on Circumcision, April 30–May 3, San Francisco, California.

Parfit, D. 1984. *Reasons and persons*. Oxford: Clarendon Press.

Patel, H. 1966. The problem of routine circumcision. *Canadian Medical Association Journal* 95: 576–81.

Penn, J. 1963. Penile reform. *British Journal of Plastic Surgery* 16: 287–88.

Puzella, C. 1997. Abortion rights of minors, parental consent and parental notification. *Journal of Contemporary Legal Issues* 11 (642): 642–47.

Ray, M. G. 1997. Like father, like son. http://www.mothersagainstcirc.org/Like-Son.htm.

Ross, L. F. 1993. Moral grounding for the participation of children as organ donors. *Journal of Law, Medicine & Ethics* 21 (2): 251–57.

Simpson, E. T. 1998. The management of the paediatric foreskin. *Australian Family Physician* 27 (5): 381–83.

# 3

## ✢

# Genital Alteration of Female Minors

## *Dena S. Davis*

It is now illegal in the United States to perform genital alteration on female minors, no matter how minimal the surgery or how safe and sanitary the procedure. Newborn male genital alteration, however, is an accepted procedure in the United States. The law takes no cognizance of the male procedure, with no records kept of circumcisions performed outside of hospitals, and with no oversight or licensing of ritual practitioners.

Why does the law turn a blind eye to one procedure and criminalize the other? Two possible answers present themselves. Part of the answer points to the relatively minor and low-risk character of newborn male circumcision, contrasted to the pain, suffering, morbidity, and death associated with female genital alteration. With regard to the most common practices of female alteration, this is a good answer. The practice as carried out in most countries well deserves the name "female genital mutilation." It is emphatically not my goal here to defend that practice nor to weaken the international movement to eradicate it. However, the federal and state laws criminalizing genital alteration on female minors are so broad that they cover even procedures significantly less substantial than newborn male circumcision. One consequence of these laws' wide sweep is that they block the efforts of compassionate and creative physicians who want to attempt to offer a compromise to immigrant parents from countries where female genital alteration is the norm. By offering a tiny, safe procedure, these physicians hope to dissuade parents from sending their girls back to Africa for the procedure or from employing a local traditional practitioner.

When one begins to question the normative status of male newborn alteration in the West, and when one thinks of female alteration as including even a hygienically administered "nick," one sees that these two practices—dramatically separated in the public imagination—actually have significant areas of overlap. Elsewhere, I have shown that the two practices lack a legally defensible distinction, given the current wording of state and federal statutes (Davis 2001). Thus, a complete laissez-faire attitude toward one practice, coupled with total criminalization of the other, runs afoul of the "free exercise" clause of the First Amendment. There are also troubling implications for the constitutional requirement of equal protection, because the laws appear to protect little girls, but not little boys, from religious and culturally motivated surgery.

## FEMALE GENITAL ALTERATION

### Description and Epidemiology

The scope and consequences of female genital alteration (FGA) have been well rehearsed in the legal and medical literature. The practice affects between 80 million and 110 million women now living worldwide, especially, but not exclusively, in Muslim cultures (Dorkenoo 1996, 142). Annually, FGA is performed on about 4 million to 5 million female infants and girls, most commonly on children between the ages of 4 and 10 (American Academy of Pediatrics 1998, 153).

Although taxonomies differ, the American Academy of Pediatrics categorizes FGA into four general types:

- Type I, often called "clitoridectomy," involves excision of the skin around the clitoris. It may also involve excision of all or part of the clitoris.
- Type II, called "excision," involves the removal of the entire clitoris and part or all of the labia minora. Bleeding from this procedure may be staunched with stitches of catgut or thorns; mud poultices may be applied directly to the wound.
- In Type III, known as "infibulation," the girl not only loses her clitoris and labia minora, but the outer labia are first cut and then stitched together, to create a permanent closure with only a small opening for urine and menstrual flow. Women who have been subjected to this procedure must then be cut open before intercourse, and require episiotomies to avoid tearing of the vulva during childbirth. (This is also sometimes referred to as "pharaonic circumcision.")
- Category IV is a catch-all covering other kinds of procedures of various degrees of severity, including piercing of the clitoris or labia, cauterization of the clitoris, and so on (1998, 153–54).

As would be expected given the medically primitive conditions in which FGA commonly takes place, the physical consequences can be horrendous. Bleeding to death is the most tragic result of the procedure; no statistics exist as to how often this takes place. Other immediate complications include shock, hemorrhage, infection, damage to the urethra or anus, scarring, and tetanus. The use of unsterilized instruments also provides a pathway for infection from bloodborne viruses such as hepatitis-B and HIV (American Medical Association 1995, 1714–15).

There are long-term health risks as well. New opportunities for infection occur when the scar tissue on infibulated women is opened when they marry or give birth. Tightly infibulated women can only urinate drop by drop, so that it can take between ten and fifteen minutes to void the bladder. Long-term complications of even the less extensive procedures include chronic vaginal, bladder, and uterine infections (often leading to sterility). When infibulated women give birth, failure to cut the scar open in time can lead to fetal damage and death (American Medical Association 1995, 1714–15). The very high rates of infant and maternal death in Sudan and Somalia are likely due in part to the fact that FGA in those countries is almost universal (Lane and Rubinstein 1996, 35).

## Alternatives to Female Genital Alteration

Because the cultural meaning of the female ritual surgery is complex and multilayered, there is hope that the procedure can be eradicated gradually by finding less harmful ways to fulfill the same functions. For example, many commentators, from both within and without societies that practice female ritual surgeries, note that the practice serves to bond women together and to cement their identities as members of the group.[1] In cultures where the ritual is practiced on older girls, it is seen as the doorway into adulthood (Teare 1998). Thus, some indigenous work against the practice has shown progress by substituting other rituals, or at least by lessening the severity of the procedure.

As an example of the latter, Gruenbaum describes what she observed in villages in the Sudan in the 1970s and 1980s. In northern Sudan, FGA was virtually universal in the 1980s. The most severe form, the "pharaonic," involving total excision of the clitoris, prepuce, labia minora, and labia majora followed by infibulation, was practiced by the majority ethnic group, the Kenana. Others practiced an "intermediate" form, and a small minority, the Zabarma, practiced the "Sunna" form, involving clitoridectomy or partial clitoridectomy only (Gruenbaum 1996, 458). By 1989, Gruenbaum observed a significant shift from the more severe to less destructive form of the procedure, due to individuals and organizations within Sudan who had spoken out against the pharaonic practice.

In Wad Medani, an old city on the west bank of the Blue Nile, the capital of Gezira Province, Gruenbaum interviewed a nurse-midwife, Sister Battool.

> Sister Battool is a renowned nurse-midwife who supports the public health education efforts to inform people about the dangers of the pharaonic form and trains other health workers. Sister Battool reported having considerable success in influencing her clients to opt for minimal tissue removal, success that she attributed to changing social attitudes. . . . For those parents who insisted on infibulation, she tried to preserve the clitoris and erectile tissue inside, so as to minimize bleeding and preserve sexual sensitivity. (1996, 469)

Another healthworker, a female physician, has become convinced through study of Islamic texts that no type of FGA is religiously required. However, she observed that the policy of the Sudanese Ministry of Health, which was against any form of the procedure, had met with such widespread popular opposition that she saw no hope for its adoption. Her strategy was to become an advocate for the least destructive form of the surgery, removing only the clitoral prepuce. "That procedure, she felt, might satisfy people's desire to circumcise, yet would leave the clitoris better exposed to sexual stimulation and improve women's sexual response" (470).

In Kenya, the rate of FGA has dropped substantially. In 1991, a survey of adolescents found that 78 percent of them had undergone the procedure, compared to 100 percent of women over the age of 50. A novel alternative rite, involving 13 rural communities as of 1998, is worth describing at length. This rite is called *Ntanira Na Mugambo*, "circumcision through words." Because the key to success is to involve the girl's family and community, the rite is flexible enough to change from one community to another; female adolescents, family members, and others in the community participate in designing the ceremony. There is also a "family life" educational component in the schools, and a program targeting young males, explaining to them the health risks women face as a result of FGA and enlisting them in a process that ends with making a vow not to require that their future wives be circumcised. The rite itself typically involves a week of seclusion for the adolescent girls, where they are taught about sexual and reproductive health, bodily anatomy, respect for adults, how to withstand peer pressure, and so on. The week ends with a public celebration in which the girls are the center of attention, receive gifts, and are given certificates. "Because the rite does not exert a blunt prohibition on female genital mutilation being practised in Kenya, but offers an attractive alternative, it is possible that it may become the most successful strategy towards more widespread elimination throughout the world" (Chelala 1998, 126).

In Israel, where Bedouin tribes already practice an extremely mild type of FGA, it has been suggested that the World Health Organization "train medical-religious functionaries to perform a sterile minor incision and then declare [that the] girl [has been] circumcised" (Cohen-Almagor 1996, 177).

In Indonesia, genital cuttings used to occur but are no longer performed. What persists, for some people, is a ritual form of the practice, consisting of cleaning the clitoris with herbal juice, a symbolic scratch of the girls' labia majora, or a "light puncture of the clitoris" (World Health Organization 1998, 21).

Accounts exist of women who only pretend to circumcise girls. An African mother says:

> Everyone tries to persuade me that it must be done to my daughter, saying that no one will marry her, but I tell them I don't care. Let her get old enough to decide what she wants for herself. In a year or so I will have a party for her and pretend that I am going to circumcise her. I will buy her new clothes, paint her hands with henna, and call in the midwife, exactly as I would if I were to have her circumcised. Then I will pay the midwife to do nothing, and tell everyone that it has been done. (Lewis 1995, 26)

In Guinea, the chief practitioner of FGA was Aja Toun-kara Diallo Fatimata, who was reviled by Western human rights activists. However, she recently confessed that she had never actually cut anyone. "I'd just pinch their clitorises to make them scream . . . and tightly bandage them up so that they walked as though they were in pain" (*Economist* 1999).

## THE LEGAL SITUATION IN THE UNITED STATES

In 1997, Representative Pat Schroeder (D-Colo.) finally succeeded in having opposition to FGA on minors encoded in the criminal law. With a couple of minor exemptions to address situations of medical necessity (e.g., deinfibulation of women in childbirth), the law states:

> . . . whoever knowingly circumcises, excises, or infibulates the whole or any part of the labia majora or labia minora or clitoris of another person who has not attained the age of 18 years shall be fined under this title or imprisoned not more than 5 years, or both. . . .
>
> No account shall be taken of the effect on the person on whom the operation is to be performed of any belief on the part of that person, or any other person, that the operation is required as a matter of custom or ritual.

The 1995 version of the Act (H.R. 941) had directed the Secretary of Health and Human Services to compile data on females, both adults and minors, living in the United States who have been subjected to the surgery and to carry out outreach and educational initiatives to those communities within the United States who traditionally practice the custom, but that provision did not survive. However, the 1997 version is partnered with a law requiring the Immigration and Naturalization Service to hand out materials on the ill effects and legal consequences of female genital mutilation to immigrants from countries where it is commonly practiced.[2]

At least 15 states have criminalized female genital mutilation, and Illinois, Minnesota, Rhode Island, and Tennessee prohibit the practice on adult women as well as minors (Rahman and Toubia 2000, 120–21)—giving rise to provocative questions about why other forms of cosmetic surgery, such as breast enlargement, are not within the purview of the law (Sheldon and Wilkinson 1988, 263). Six states explicitly hold parents or legal guardians of minors criminally liable if they consent to or initiate the procedure (Rahman and Toubia 2000).

Although most state laws track the language of the federal statute, some, such as North Dakota, give a more explicitly sweeping description of what constitutes the criminal act: "Any person who knowingly separates or surgically alters normal, healthy, functioning genital tissue of a female minor is guilty of a class C felony" (Key 1997, 179–80).

## THE SEATTLE EXPERIENCE

In 1996, physicians at Harborview Medical Center in Seattle decided to try a novel approach to save young girls from the horrors of traditional genital alteration. Doctors and nurses in obstetrical practice had been startled by pregnant Somali women who, when asked if they wanted their baby circumcised if it was a boy, responded, "Yes, and also if it's a girl."[3] In addition, Somali mothers were asking physicians to perform minimalist procedures on their adolescent daughters' genitals. The women explained that, if they could not have some form of the procedure done safely in the United States, they would take their girls back to Somalia, where in all likelihood they would be subjected to the most severe procedure,[4] or have the procedure done in the United States by an imported traditional practitioner.[5]

The idea of a symbolic cut, a tiny bloodletting under hygienic conditions with no foreseeable sequelae, came initially from the Somali women themselves. The hospital was intrigued by a possible compromise that offered a way out of a terrible dilemma; refusing to do the procedure simply condemned the girls to an uncontrolled, unsupervised, life-threatening array of possibilities in their homeland. According to the compromise, girls old enough to provide consent[6] would undergo a tiny nick on the prepuce, which would be performed with appropriate analgesia and under sterile conditions.[7] The operation would be less extensive than the commonly practiced male circumcision, more analogous to ear piercing. The community-bonding, cultural aspects of the practice would be preserved, as the girls' mothers would be able to invite the community to the hospital, organize appropriate rituals, throw a party to honor the girls, and so on.[8]

Harborview's experiment never got off the ground, however. The hospital administration, as well as individual doctors, received hate mail and death threats; accounts in the press were uniformly unsympathetic and usually lurid. What is most interesting about this story are the legal ramifications of Harborview's proposed experiment. At the time of the public brouhaha, the federal law authored by Representative Schroeder had been passed but had not yet taken effect. Schroeder herself wrote to Harborview, saying that she believed the proposal would violate the new law.[9] "The clear intent of the legislation," she wrote, "was to criminalize any medically unnecessary procedure involving female genitalia" (Coleman 1998, 752). Certainly, under some forms of state criminal statutes, such as North Dakota's, any practice, no matter how minimal, would constitute a felony under the "surgically alters" wording of the law.

The Seattle experience makes clear that, at least in the eyes of the federal law's primary author, even a tiny cut with proper medical precautions done on a minor female's genitalia is illegal. Male circumcision, however, which is a more substantial procedure than the one contemplated in Seattle, is legal even when done by traditional, nonmedical practitioners in the home. The comparison between male circumcision and female genital mutilation, while "usually disingenuous," in this case was "ultimately legitimate" (Coleman 1998, 736).

## DISCUSSION

FGA does not bring any health benefits. In the Third World countries where most FGA takes place, it is associated with horrendous risk of death and serious complications, even into maturity. It is usually performed without pain control, and young girls are often emotionally traumatized. When FGA is performed in the West, its illicit and "back room" nature makes it reasonable to assume that the risks remain very high. With the exception of the small nick proposed in Seattle, all forms of FGA remove substantial parts of a woman's sexual organs. The effect on the subjects' sexuality, while not adequately studied, is clearly negative. The procedure can be understood as gender subjugation, as a rite of passage to maturity and membership in the group, or as a sign of female independence and self-respect, as some practitioners and supporters insist. The reasons why parents subject their daughters to FGA include a mix of religion, custom, group cohesion, concern for cultural survival, family pressure, a misunderstanding of medical benefits, and economic concerns.

Male genital alteration's (MGA) health benefits are controversial and attenuated. No major medical group currently supports the practice of MGA. Despite clear calls for pain control from, for example, the American Academy of Pediatrics (AAP), fewer than half of baby boys receive adequate analgesia. The risks of death and serious complications appear quite small, although better data are needed. Although MGA removes less tissue than most forms of FGA, some scientists argue that the foreskin is a substantial factor in sexual feeling and behavior. MGA removes significantly more tissue than the "nick" proposed in Seattle. The effect on the subjects' sexuality has not been adequately studied, but there is some evidence to suggest that it is negative. For Americans who are neither Jews nor Muslims, the procedure is purely a matter of aesthetics and custom or some generally misunderstood view of the supposed health benefits. For religious Jews, it is an obligation of the highest order, but the majority of American Jews do not have their sons' genital alteration performed in a ritually correct manner. The procedure can be understood variably as deeply sexist, as a celebration of group identity and cultural survival, as anti-erotic, and as a rite of passage. The reasons why parents subject their sons to MGA include religion, custom, group cohesion, family pressure, a misunderstanding of medical benefits, and economic motivations from those who perform circumcisions (Davis 2001).

At the present time, MGA is no longer considered routine, has no strong medical benefit, and is a decision made by parents largely on religious and cultural grounds. MGA is legal in this country, with no oversight, whether it is practiced by physicians or by traditional *mohels*. FGA, on the other hand, a decision also made by parents on religious and cultural grounds, is illegal even if its actual expression is a ritual nick of less physical import and carrying less risk than the traditional male procedure. What this boils down to is, if you are an American Jew, you can have your baby boy genitally altered with impunity, even if it is done outside a hospital by an unlicensed ritual practitioner, and without the analgesia deemed "essential" by the AAP.[10] But if you are a recent immigrant from Somalia, even if you would take the enlightened route and subject your daughter to a ritual nick at the Seattle clinic, you (and the doctor) would be subject to criminal prosecution. This is unacceptable on First Amendment grounds.

We may imagine male and female genital alterations as two circles with some degree of overlap. Although there are many important differences between the two practices, there is clearly an area where the risks of harm to the child are substantially the same. Indeed, if we compare the Seattle proposal to the unregulated practice of traditional *berit mila* (ritual Jewish circumcision of newborn males), it appears that the latter involves more skin removed, with less likelihood of adequate pain control and no systematic reporting system for complications. The Seattle proposal was "less injurious to the health, welfare and safety of girls than male circumcision is to the health, welfare and safety of boys" (Coleman 1998, 761). The primary difference between the operation proposed in Seattle (as well as some extremely minor forms of FGA already in practice) and the one performed daily on newborn males in America is that the first is associated with "bizarre" practices brought to America by strange people practicing strange customs, while the other is a Western practice with which we are comfortable and familiar. Of course, another important difference, which I will address below, is that the circle comprising all of FGA includes much more horrible practices, both quantitatively and qualitatively.

If then, we "match up" a deeply religious Muslim couple who wish to have their daughter altered, who believe it is a religious obligation, and who are willing to accept the Seattle compromise, with a deeply religious Jewish couple who wish to have their son altered because they believe it is a religious obligation, it is hard to justify why the first couple's wish is illegal and the second's is not. If we imagine that the Muslim girl's experience will be a tiny nick with proper pain control in a hospital context, while the Jewish boy's experience will be a somewhat larger operation by a nonmedical practitioner without adequate pain control, the justification becomes even more difficult.

The best argument in defense of laws criminalizing FGA is that allowing even the benign Seattle compromise will handicap health and government workers in stamping out the more horrible forms of this practice. Because FGA in its most common forms around the world is mutilating and life threatening, it is reasonable to adopt a "zero tolerance policy" to make it absolutely clear to immigrants that this practice is never acceptable. When the debate became public in Seattle, a number of activists, including those from cultures where FGA is the rule, protested that offering any form of FGA would seriously dilute their efforts to educate immigrant parents. Further, an argument could be made that, once a "nick" is allowed, it would be difficult if not impossible for the state to make sure that this did not become a loophole through which the worst elements of FGA would slide.[11] As MGA is not anywhere close to as mutilating and threatening to life and health as are many forms of FGA, this argument would serve as a valid distinction between the two practices.

However, a number of commentators have made the point that allowing something like the Seattle compromise would strengthen, not weaken, the ability of educators to persuade immigrants away from their traditional FGA practices. A willingness to compromise would show respect for the immigrants' culture and religion and would exhibit tolerance within the necessary limits of protecting children against abuse (Coleman 1998, 773). The fact that a significant number of Somali women were willing to take up Harborview Hospital's offer suggests that the "ritual nick" could have become an important tool in educating the immigrant community and in giving parents an alternative to sending their girls back to Somalia or hiring a backstreet traditional practitioner.

Further, as long as the United States continues to countenance MGA, the criminalization of even the "ritual nick" cannot fail to dilute the persuasiveness of the official stance against FGA, while carrying the unmistakable taint of intolerance and double standards. It is helpful to remember how the

Seattle story began: with cognitive dissonance on both sides, as doctors routinely asked patients if they wanted their newborn boys circumcised, and patients (routinely!) answered that yes, they wanted both their boys and their girls circumcised. "Female circumcision will never stop as long as male circumcision is going on. How do you expect to convince an African father to leave his daughter uncircumcised as long as you let him do it to his son?" (Abu-Sahlieh 1994).

## CONCLUSION AND RECOMMENDATIONS

Doriane Lambelet Coleman asserts:

> A state such as Washington has two options. It can begin performing symbolic female circumcisions, or it can stop circumcising or condoning the circumcision of boys. While the latter option would immediately raise substantial and very legitimate First Amendment concerns for parents whose religion requires circumcision—concerns that could be articulated just as easily by parents of boys and girls—it is clear that the choice must be made one way or the other. The bottom line is that the state cannot treat parents differently on the basis of their child's gender. (1998, 766)

Nor, I would add, can a state or the federal government treat parents differently on the basis of their differing religious beliefs.

Facing up to the religious discrimination inherent in the current legal state of affairs is a good beginning. Just acknowledging that the complex, fuzzy reasons why a secular Jew would alter her son are no more or less worthy of respect than the complex, fuzzy reasons why a Somali mother would alter her daughter, is an important first step. Beyond that, I make the following recommendations. These recommendations are a compromise that seeks to protect young girls and boys from traumatic genital alteration, while respecting the important motivations that underlie both FGA and MGA. Further, by closing somewhat the gap between the total legal condemnation of any form of FGA and the complete legal indifference to MGA, these recommendations will go some way toward showing respect for immigrants from cultures that practice FGA and removing the taint of religious intolerance.

1. Federal and state laws should be rewritten to allow the sort of minor genital nick, with proper pain control and in hygienic circumstances, contemplated by Harborview General Hospital. (Of course, this would not obligate health care providers to offer that service.)
2. States should exercise some control over the practice of MGA when performed without medical necessity on minors.
3. States should gather data on all MGA, whether or not it is performed in the hospital, and whether or not the practitioner is a physician. All com-

plications of MGA should be reported, to allow for a better understanding of the medical implications of this practice and also to allow
oversight of nonmedical practitioners.
4. Nonphysician ritual practitioners of MGA should be certified. At present, this is probably the most serious operation one can perform without being charged with practicing medicine without a license. While requiring a medical license might well be overkill, requiring some sort of
board certification, effected by the religious community but with government oversight, seems reasonable. The state regulates the hygienic
practices of the people who cut our hair and our fingernails, so why not
a baby's genitals?
5. Adequate pain control should be a legal requirement. Failure to provide it, within a clinical or a traditional setting, should be considered
grounds for child abuse.

In conclusion, it has not been my goal to soften or subvert the opposition
to FGA of minors. However, a close look at the suggested Seattle compromise and its outcome shows us that there is significant overlap between
some forms of FGA and the common practice of MGA in America. But one
practice is illegal, while the other is not even the object of governmental
oversight or record-keeping. Analysis of the motives behind the two
practices—religious, medical, cultural, social—do not support such a disparity. The rhetoric of the activists, and the language of the federal and state
laws against FGA, all suggest that this disparity is driven at least in part by
a deep lack of respect for motivations that drive parents to perform FGA, as
contrasted with the respect given the motivations behind MGA. In the recommendations above, I suggest a number of steps to address the disparity
of treatment, while strengthening society's proper concern for the health and
welfare of all children.

## NOTES

1. Bonnie Shullenberger, "Africans view circumcision as rite," *New York Times*, June 22, 1995.
Shullenberger observes, "Circumcision in both males and females in Africa is a mark of cultural
identity; it designates one's membership in one's tribe and participation in its life and assumptions."
2. 8 U.S.C.A. § 1374 (West 1999).
3. Tom Brune, "Refugees' beliefs don't travel well; Compromise plan on circumcision of
girls gets little support," *Chicago Tribune*, October 28, 1996.
4. Carol M. Ostrom, "Harborview debates issue of circumcision of Muslim girls," *Seattle
Times*, September 13, 1996.
5. Lisa M. Hamm, "Immigrants bring the practice of female circumcision to the U.S.," Associated Press, November 18, 1996.
6. I share with the reader a grave doubt about the validity of this consent, given everything that has been said about the pervasiveness of this custom and the dreadful life

prospects imagined for girls who do not have some form of the procedure done. In my view, the "consent" requirement was just window dressing.

7. Brune, "Refugees' beliefs don't travel well."

8. Telephone conversation with Leslie R. Miller, assistant professor of obstetrics/gynecology, Harborview Medical Center, Seattle, Washington.

9. Celia W. Dugger, "Tug of taboos: African genital rite vs. U.S. law," *New York Times*, December 28, 1996. It remains somewhat unclear whether Schroeder had all the facts when she made that pronouncement. It is also unclear whether the compromise, had it been implemented, would have run afoul of state laws against child abuse.

10. Despite documented cases of transmission of herpes simplex virus by mohels who continue to use direct oral–genital contact to suction blood from the circumcision wound, some ultra-Orthodox mohels and rabbis continue to support the practice. Officials at Agudath Israel, which is headed by a council of ultra-Orthodox rabbis, have defended the practice, which was publicly condemned in 2004 by modern Orthodox rabbi and scientist Moshe Tendler (Steven I. Weiss, "Rabbi targeted after call for bris change," *Forward*, March 18, 2005. See also Gesundheit et al. 2004.

11. Justice Sandra Day O'Connor made this argument with respect to Oregon's law criminalizing even the religious use of peyote: "[I]n view of the societal interest in preventing trafficking in controlled substances, uniform application of the criminal prohibition at issue is essential to the effectiveness of Oregon's stated interest in preventing any possession of peyote." *Employment Div.* v. *Smith*, 494 U.S. 872, 905 (1990) (O'Connor, J., concurring).

# REFERENCES

Abu-Sahlieh, Sami A. Aldeeb. 1994. To mutilate in the name of Jehovah or Allah: Legitimization of male and female circumcision. *Medicine & Law* 13 (7–8): 575–622.

American Academy of Pediatrics, Committee on Bioethics. 1998. Female genital mutilation. *Pediatrics* 102: 153.

American Medical Association, Council on Scientific Affairs. 1995. Female genital mutilation. *Journal of the American Medical Association* 274: 1714–15.

Chelala, Cesar. 1998. An alternative way to stop female genital mutilation. *Lancet* 352: 126.

Cohen-Almagor, Raphael. 1996. Female circumcision and murder for family honour among minorities in Israel. In *Nationalism, Minorities and Diasporas: Identities and Rights in the Middle East*, ed. Kirsten E. Schulze, Martin Stokes, and Colm Campbell. London: Tauris Academic Studies.

Coleman, Dorian Lambelet. 1998. The Seattle compromise: Multicultural sensitivity and Americanization. *Duke Law Journal* 47: 717–83.

Davis, Dena S. 2001. Male and female genital alteration: A collision course with the law? *Health Matrix* 11: 487–570.

Dorkenoo, Efua. 1996. Combating female genital mutilation: An agenda for the next decade. *World Health Statistics Quarterly* 49: 142–47.

*Economist*. 1999. Female genital mutilation: Is it crime or culture? *Economist*, February 13.

Gesundheit, Benjamin, et al. Neonatal genetal herpes simplex virus type 1 infection after Jewish ritual circumcision: Modern medicine and religious tradition. 2004. *Pediatrics* 114 (2): 259–63.

Gruenbaum, Ellen. 1996. The cultural debate over female circumcision. The Sudanese are arguing this one out for themselves. *Medical Anthropology Quarterly* 10 (4): 455–75.

Key, Frances L. 1997. Female circumcision/female genital mutilation in the United States: Legislation and its implications for health providers. *Journal of the American Medical Women's Association* 52: 179–81.

Lane, Sandra D., and Robert A. Rubinstein. 1996. Judging the other: Responding to traditional female genital surgeries. *Hastings Center Report* 26 (3): 31–40.

Lewis, Hope. 1995. Between Irua and "Female Genital Mutilation:" Feminist Human Rights Discourse and the Cultural Divide. *Harvard Human Rights Journal* 8: 1–55.

Rahman, Anika, and Nahid Toubia, eds. 2000. *Female genital mutilation: A guide to laws and policies worldwide*. London: Zed Books.

Sheldon, Sally, and Stephen Wilkinson. 1988. Female genital mutilation and cosmetic surgery: Regulating non-therapeutic body modification. *Bioethics* 12: 263–85.

Teare, Parasathi. 1998. Hot potatoes. *Nursing Times* 94 (49): 32–34.

World Health Organization. 1998. *Female genital mutilation: An overview*, prepared by Nahid Toubia and Susan Izett. Geneva: World Health Organization.

# II

# SEX ASSIGNMENT AND REASSIGNMENT SURGERY

The Ethics of Surgically Assigning Sex for Intersex Children
*Merle Spriggs and Julian Savulescu*

Transsexualism and Gender Reassignment Surgery
*Heather Draper and Neil Evans*

# 4

## ✛

# The Ethics of Surgically Assigning Sex for Intersex Children

### *Merle Spriggs and Julian Savulescu*

Intersex conditions raise profound ethical issues for the children born with these conditions, for their parents and for clinicians. *Intersex* refers to conditions "in which chromosomal sex is inconsistent with phenotypic sex, or in which the phenotype is not classifiable as either male or female" (Sax 2002, 174). This means that a child with an intersex condition may be genetically female with external genitalia that appear to be male, or may be genetically male with external genitalia that appear to be female. In some rare cases the child has both male and female genitalia. The prevalence of these conditions is 1.8 in every 10,000 live births, and the most common of the "classic intersex conditions" are congenital adrenal hyperplasia (CAH) and complete androgen insensitivity syndrome (CAIS) (Sax 2002, 174–75). There is debate about the definition of *intersex*. Broader definitions, of course, will give a higher prevalence (Blackless et al. 2000).

In this chapter, our concern is with the contentious issue of early surgery—situations where the surgical assignment of sex or "corrective" surgery is an option. In the literature and in practice guidelines, intersex conditions are variously referred to as "developmental anomalies of the external genitalia" (American Academy of Pediatrics 2000), "atypical sexual differentiation" (Cohen-Kettenis and Pfäfflin 2003), and "ambiguous genitalia" (Rangecroft 2003; Low, Hutson, and Murdoch Childrens Research Institute Sex Study Group 2003), even though intersex children "may or may not be born with external genitals that are ambiguous" (Cohen-Kettenis and Pfäfflin 2003, 49). Some intersex conditions remain undetected until puberty or later.

Intersex conditions can be harmful in three ways. First, the condition itself can be harmful. The range of intersex condition may include recurrent urinary tract infections (Warne 2003), problems with infertility, precocious or delayed puberty, hormonal imbalance requiring medication, risk of cancer, problems with sexual functioning and satisfaction, and gender identity and relationship difficulties leading to social and psychological problems (Cohen-Kettenis and Pfäfflin 2003, 90–91). Second, openness about an infant's condition in an environment where people are not aware of, don't understand, and don't accept genital ambiguity can lead to the child being stigmatized. Third, not disclosing the child's condition creates "an atmosphere of secrecy" suggesting that the child suffers from "something shameful" (Cohen-Kettenis and Pfäfflin 2003, 87–88). The attitude that ambiguous genitals are shameful is a "primary source of harm" for people with intersex conditions (Chase 1998).

Standard medical practice has been to make an early diagnosis and to perform early "corrective" genital surgery. The reasoning behind this is the need for a clear and unambiguous sex assignment to save intersex children from being ostracized and to enable parents to bond with their baby girl or baby boy (American Academy of Pediatrics 2000; Lawson Wilkins Pediatric Endocrine Society and European Society for Paediatric Endocrinology 2002). The commonly described goals of such surgery are listed in box 4-1.

Types of early surgery include feminizing genitoplasty, which involves the removal of tissue from what is either an enlarged clitoris or a small penis and surgery to enlarge or to create a vagina (Warne 2003). Early gonadectomy (removal of testes) is sometimes carried out because malignant change is

---

**Box 4-1.   Goals or Objectives of Early Surgery**

From various sources and perspectives the following have been identified as the goals or objectives of early surgery:

- Normal looking genitalia to encourage stable gender identity and reduce stigma and psychological distress (Paediatric Surgeons Working Party 2001, appendix [referring to practice based on the work of John Money])
- Pediatric urologists want to provide the patient with positive psychosocial and psychosexual adjustments throughout life (Schober 2004, 698)
- Patients and parents want surgery that looks cosmetically authentic and provides good function (Schober 2004, 697)
- The "psychological benefit of the parents" (Warne 2003)
- To allow the child to avoid the psychological problems from being different from other children and the "cruel discrimination" that that might bring about (Warne 2003)
- To allow the child to grow up without medical problems caused by the anatomy (Warne 2003)
- Early surgery confers some medical benefits (Warne 2003)
- To remove "anatomic or functional obstacles to the development of healthy and satisfactory sexuality" (Warne 2003)

thought to be a possibility in infants who have testes which are intra-abdominal or contained in inguinal herniae (Rangecroft 2003).

A growing number of objectors have argued against early genital surgery on the grounds that it is not necessary, is not reversible, and can cause harm (Intersex Society of North America 1998). Some commentators argue that surgery to normalize the infant is based on parents' fears and concerns rather than the best interests of the child and amounts to "the medical management of a psychological condition" performed on the child for the sake of the parents (Purves 2000, 30–37): "Cosmetic surgeries are performed without the subject's consent because of adults' discomfort with intersexuality" (Dreger 1999, 17).

The central questions in the management of intersex infants are:

- When, if ever, should surgery be carried out?
- Who should decide?
- On what criteria should decisions be based?

The focus of the above issues for some seems to be the child's future autonomy and the implications of parents or others making irrevocable decisions for young children. We will argue that the main ethical issue is not a question of autonomy but the question of whether surgery makes the child's life go better or worse. We begin by outlining the criticisms of the traditional treatment model and early surgery and then address the central questions.

## THE CHALLENGE TO THE
## TRADITIONAL TREATMENT MODEL AND EARLY SURGERY

Since the 1990s the traditional treatment model has been challenged. Opposition to "normalizing" surgery for people with intersex conditions has been expressed by patient advocacy groups and through the personal testimony of patients who are not happy with the way their condition has been managed.

Are medical professionals standing by with rulers and stamps of approval? To some extent they are, and we are all subject to their judgement. . . . We are not so quick to judge other parts of anatomy. We teach our children to respect diversity, yet adults create a "state of emergency" over the size and shape of genitals. The real phenomenon is that the prevalence of genital and reproductive variation is kept such a secret. Intersex variations are so quickly "disappeared" that we don't get a chance to know about them, or how they might mature. . . .

At the age of 13, I was scheduled for surgery. . . . My body was altered to meet social values, but my values were never discussed. My puberty was focused on vaginal function before I had a chance to care. (Morris 2004, 25–27)

One of the criticisms of the traditional treatment model is that it fails to recognize the experience of intersexed people and to recognize that they are experts in terms of their experience of intersex conditions (Dreger 1999, 19). Another factor in the opposition to early genital surgery is the failed sex reassignment of an infant whose penis was completely burned off in a circumcision accident—the much publicized "John-Joan case" (Aaronson 2004).

In this case, a biologically unambiguous male infant was reassigned to the female sex on the recommendation of psychologist John Money, who claimed that infants are sexually neutral, that nurture trumps nature, and that gender identity is determined by the prenatal environment (Daaboul and Frader 2001). In a series of publications, Money reported that the surgically reassigned male infant had been successfully reared as a girl—resulting in the wide dissemination of the view that gender is malleable. He wrote that "no one" would "ever conjecture" that the child was born a boy (Kipnis and Diamond 1998, 176). Ultimately, however, gender reassignment in this case proved unsuccessful. The child "never became a normal girl" and from the age of 14 lived as a male (Kipnis and Diamond 1998, 180). He underwent four rounds of reconstructive surgery and in 2004, at the age of 38, he committed suicide.[1] Many have taken this case as evidence that the claim that gender is socially constructed is wrong (Aaronson 2004).

In relation to the surgical assignment of sex, Kipnis and Diamond (1998, 186–88) make three recommendations which have wide support among those who oppose early surgery:

1. "That there be a general moratorium on such surgery when it is done without the consent of the patient." Kipnis and Diamond argue that doctors should not perform the surgery without the knowledge that "comparable patients generally do badly without the surgery." They also argue that the lack of evidence about benefits means that surgical assignment of sex is an "experimental procedure." Their objection is to the "*surgical* assignment of sex, not to gender assignment per se."

2. "That this moratorium not be lifted unless and until the medical profession completes comprehensive look-back studies and finds that the outcomes of past interventions have been positive." Kipnis and Diamond claim that retrospective outcome studies can be done with the thousands of grown intersexuals who have and have not had surgical and hormonal treatment.

3. "That efforts be made to undo the effects of past deception by physicians."

## WHO SHOULD DECIDE?

One of the controversies about early genital surgery focuses on the question of who should decide or who should have the authority to consent to surgery on behalf of children with intersex conditions. Should parents, doctors, or the courts decide, or should the decision be left to children themselves when they become old enough?

Parents are usually the best placed to judge what is in their children's best interests and ordinarily have authority to make medical decisions for them. However, there are some medical procedures for which parental consent is considered insufficient. These include interventions which are grave and irreversible, involve significant risk, involve difficult ethical issues, or are not for the purpose of treating an illness. Such interventions sometimes require court authorization.

In Australia there is a legal category of "special medical procedures" that require authorization. These procedures include nontherapeutic sterilization and hysterectomy, gender reassignment, and organ donation. The Australian High Court decided that some grave and irreversible medical procedures that may permanently affect a child's quality of life are not within the scope of parents' or guardians' powers and should be made by "an objective, independent umpire" such as the Family Court (Family Court of Australia 1998, vii).[2] The High Court thought that special medical procedures require special consideration because there is a significant risk of making a wrong decision and grave consequences for the child would follow if a wrong decision were made (2). Consideration of the child's best interests, using factors listed in box 4-2, was one of the key issues identified by the court.

Surgery for intersex newborns and infants falls into the category of special medical procedures requiring court authorization because it is irreversible, involves risk, and sometimes—namely, when the aim is for the genitals to match the assigned gender—is performed for cosmetic reasons rather than to treat an illness.

While it is generally assumed that parents will act in the best interests of their children, courts will scrutinize parents' decisions about their children's

---

**Box 4-2.  Factors Taken into Account in Assessing a Child's Best Interests**

- The difficulties facing the child and family that led to the treatment being proposed
- The attitude of the child and parent or custodian to the proposed procedure and to any alternative medical procedures or options
- Weighing up the advantages and disadvantages of the procedure and any available alternatives
- Assessing the nature and degree of risk to the child from the procedure and the alternatives
- Assessing whether the procedure needs to happen now or whether other options can be tested and, if unsuccessful, the procedure can be performed in the future (Family Court of Australia 1998, 24–25)

medical treatments when it seems they are not acting in their child's best interests or if they have a conflict of interest. Some people think that parents
choosing surgery for their intersex infants involves a conflict of interest
in the sense that it is difficult for parents to be sure that they are acting in
their child's best interests when they are being pressured to make a quick
decision.

The first high court in the world to consider the question of whether parents should or should not have the authority to choose surgery for their intersex children was the Constitutional Court of Colombia (Greenberg and
Chase n.d.). The court decided in 1999 that "under the then existing medical
practices in Colombia" parents might not be "in the best position" to make
medical decisions for their intersex children for the following reasons:

1. parents typically lack information about intersexuality;
2. intersexuality is viewed as a disease that must be "cured"; and
3. the treating physicians convey a sense of urgency to provide a quick cure.
   (Greenberg 2003, 283)

This suggests that the court was taking the view that intersexuality is not a
disease and that there is no urgency to fix the problem surgically. The court
also thought that parents "may be motivated by their own concerns and
fears rather than the 'best interests' of their children" (283).

The court carried out "exhaustive consultations" for more than a year,
hearing evidence in support of both the traditional treatment model and alternative treatment recommendations. After hearing all the evidence, the
court concluded that

> to prohibit surgeries until the children reach the age of consent would be en-
> gaging in social experimentation, but to allow the surgeries to continue under
> the standard protocol would not ensure that the best interests of the children are
> protected. (Greenberg 2003, 279)

While the court did not rule against surgery, it established rules *restricting*
parents' authority to authorize surgery (Greenberg and Chase n.d.). It recommended a new category of consent in order to make parents "put their
children's best interests ahead of their own fears and concerns about sexual
ambiguity" (Greenberg 2003, 279). The court required consent to be "qualified and persistent" and required the development of procedures by legal
and medical institutions to meet the following conditions:

1. The consent must be in writing.
2. The information provided must be complete. The parents must be informed
   about the dangers of current treatments, the existence of other paradigms,
   and the possibility of delaying surgeries and giving adequate psychological
   support to the child.

3. The authorization must be given on several occasions over a reasonable time period to make sure the parents have enough time to truly understand the situation.[3]

Some medical procedures are indeed special, requiring much thought and sometimes legal scrutiny. Based on these decisions, we should conclude that parents should ordinarily decide but the courts should be involved when a particular decision to perform surgery on an intersex child appears to be against that child's interests. This would involve someone seeking court intervention because of the belief that the child's best interests were not being served. Alternatively, surgery for intersex conditions could be classed as a "special medical procedure" requiring court authorization. Having to go to court to get authorization for surgical treatment could be traumatic for parents, but some parents may find welcome relief in sharing the weight of the decision. Next we summarize clinical guidance in these complex decisions.

## THE CLINICAL PERSPECTIVE:
## SHOULD EARLY SURGERY BE CARRIED OUT?

### Current Practice Guidelines for the Surgical Management of Intersex Newborns

*American Academy of Pediatrics*

The guidelines of the American Academy of Pediatrics (2000) famously begin with the statement: "The birth of a child with ambiguous genitalia constitutes a social emergency" (138). They emphasize the urgency of a prompt definitive diagnosis and treatment: "It is important that a definitive diagnosis be determined as quickly as possible so that an appropriate treatment plan can be established to minimize medical, psychological, and social complications" (138). The point is also made that most genital abnormalities are not ambiguous in appearance and "only a minority of intersex patients have genitalia that are so ambiguous that the sex is uncertain" (139).

According to the academy, decisions about the sex of rearing should be based on fertility potential, capacity for normal sexual function, endocrine function, and testosterone imprinting (140–41). "Ongoing counseling" of parents and affected children is recommended because of "remaining uncertainties with regard to the long term psychological and physical aspects of treatment" (141). This document states that infants raised as girls "will usually require clitoral reduction" (141).

The type of evidence supporting the recommendations in this document is not stated.[4] This guideline is due to be reviewed.

*British Association of Paediatric Surgeons*

The guidance from the British Association of Paediatric Surgeons is meant to be an "evidence based summation of current thinking and suggested practice" (Paediatric Surgeons Working Party 2001). It notes the controversy relating to standard protocols, but claims that a policy of prohibiting surgery until the fully informed consent of the patient can be obtained—that is, when the child becomes "Gillick competent" (of sufficient maturity to be capable of giving independent consent during adolescence)—seems "too prescriptive" given that there are "so many specific issues related to the different diagnostic groups" (Rangecroft 2003, 799).

This guideline recommends referral to a multidisciplinary team (Rangecroft 2003) and recommends making "no assignment of gender" prior to referral (799). It suggests that where continuing pressure from parents for early corrective surgery exists, "fully informed consent" for procedures would require parents being made aware of "the possibility of non-surgical management with psychological support for the child and family" (799).

An appendix in the draft statement on clitoral surgery notes that although no data are available, clitorectomy or clitoral amputation is thought to be rarely done in the United Kingdom now, and it is presumed that clitoral recession is no longer performed, although clitoral reduction is still carried out. It notes that there are few studies looking systematically at outcome. There are also no comparative data comparing women who have undergone surgery to women who have not had surgery, even though there is an existing cohort of older patients from the United Kingdom who have not had genital surgery to compare with babies with ambiguous genitalia from the United States—almost all who have undergone genital surgery since the 1950s (Paediatric Surgeons Working Party 2001, 7–8).

*Other Guidelines*

Other guidelines and recommendations exist (Lawson Wilkins Pediatric Endocrine Society and European Society for Paediatric Endocrinology 2002; Frader et al. 2004; Eugster 2004; Daaboul and Frader 2001). The most striking conclusion from these guidelines is that recommendations are being made in the absence of long-term data about outcomes. Some evidence exists,[5] but there are serious problems with that evidence.

- The John-Joan case is not useful in terms of evidence. That case did not involve a child with an intersex condition and genital ambiguity. The child was harmed, but the real harm was caused by the botched circumcision (Mazur 2004; Bullough 2003).
- "Systematic prospective or even systematic retrospective overall outcome studies" are not available (Reiner 2004, 51).

- There are criticisms that the traditional treatment model fails to recognize the experience of intersexed people. This raises the question: "How do we know what the experience of intersexed people is?"
- It is not easy to obtain the experience of intersexed people. "Self-descriptions" of the long-term effects of reconstructive surgery and of the anomalies themselves are "rare" (Reiner 2004). According to W. G. Reiner, a urologist who has become a psychiatrist, while clinically useful studies that claim to provide overall outcomes such as health-related quality of life do exist, they are problematic—they are too narrow in scope and "too simplistic in their understanding of quality of life" and their data are difficult to interpret and not useful if there is a lack of systematization within research and clinical care (Reiner 2004, 51).
- There are doubts about the representativeness of individuals studied. Recruiting individuals from intersex support groups is thought to give a negative bias in terms of surgical management (Schober 2004, 701–2), while recruiting individuals from clinics gives a positive bias (Meyer-Bahlburg et al. 2004). We do not know the experience of those who do not take part in follow-up studies. For example, in a study of the attitude of intersex patients, it was found that most were satisfied with the management of their condition and with the gender they were assigned (Meyer-Bahlburg et al. 2004). We have to question the value of this finding, given that more than a quarter of the patients could not be contacted and nearly a quarter refused to participate.
- Small sample size is a recurrent problem.
- Some argue that "researcher bias" results when studies are not independent from treating physicians (Frader et al. 2004, 428; Eugster 2004, 428).
- The fact that surgery is better now means that retrospective studies may not be very useful.
- Studies ask superficial questions (Meyer-Bahlburg et al. 2004, 1618).
- In a review of current research relating to feminizing genitoplasty, Schober (2004, 698) claims "no definitive information is currently available regarding the 'best time' for surgical intervention" and the risk/benefit analysis has not yet been established.
- There are some studies about clitoroplasty and vaginoplasty, but little data on functional outcome available (Schober 2004, 701–2).

## THE THREAT TO FUTURE AUTONOMY

The threat to future autonomy is one of the reasons some people object to early surgery for intersex newborns. They are concerned about what happens when parents make irrevocable decisions for their children, and they worry that the intersex child's autonomy or developing autonomy will be affected by the way his or her condition is managed.

According to one commentator, "Intersexed people have their autonomy violated because their doctors and parents are allowed to make decisions about how their genitals should look" (Dreger 1999, 17). And, an adult who was born intersexed claims, "Intersexuals aren't encouraged to be autonomous. . . . Who we are is dictated to us" (Preves 1999, 56).

Intersex people who underwent surgery when they were young may have been harmed, but the harm is not to their autonomy. To begin with, very young children do not have autonomy—immaturity precludes autonomy. Nevertheless, that is not the focus of the concerns expressed above and will not eliminate worries about threats to children's autonomy. There is a need to make a distinction between two ideas:

1. The future autonomy of the child
2. The child's developing autonomy

Damage to cognitive abilities would harm the young person's developing autonomy, but the harm alluded to in the above quotes refers to a child's future autonomy and the idea that choices made by parents will close off certain options, thereby limiting the child's autonomy. This is what some commentators refer to as "a child's right to an open future" (Feinberg 1980).

Appealing to a child's future autonomy in this way is not useful. Autonomy is not just about the number of options a person has open. Although autonomy is sometimes used as a synonym for freedom or liberty, it is about more than that. A person's liberty or freedom can be affected by a reduction in options, but the availability and range of life options is not what makes a person autonomous. Autonomy is a richer concept. It is about self-rule and making decisions about how one's life should go. It is about acting or choosing in a way that reflects preferences and values and depends on a particular kind of thinking.

As long as there are basic opportunities to grow and learn, autonomy does not depend on the circumstances in which a person finds themselves. It is possible to be autonomous and make autonomous decisions within narrowed horizons and also when options are not to our liking. Autonomous decisions can be made in reduced circumstances, such as that brought about by illness (Spriggs 1998). Most important, whether or not surgery is performed, some options will be open while others irrevocably remain closed:

1. If surgery *is not* performed, the child will later have a choice of whether or not to have surgery, but no choice over whether he/she is stigmatized as an intersex child during early development.
2. If surgery *is* performed, the child will have choices opened as a result of having a more "accepted" appearance, but no choice later on whether to have surgery.

Someone with an intersex condition who has undergone surgery as an infant may be harmed by the surgery because sensation is affected, by the feeling of shame generated by having the surgery, or by being stigmatized because of their condition. That person may have different options available than if they had not had the surgery. Fertility may be affected, for example. However, their autonomy is not determined by these factors. Certainly the sex assigned will influence a person's plans and choices, but autonomy is characterized by a person's capacity to think critically about their preferences, desires, and wishes, and their "capacity to accept or attempt to change these in light of higher-order preferences and values" (Dworkin 1988, 20). In exercising that capacity, a person "defines their nature, gives meaning and coherence to their life and takes responsibility for their choices" (Spriggs 2005, 241). Ultimately, it is the result of these choices and the way they are made that determines the kind of person they become—and that may be an autonomous, mostly autonomous, sometimes autonomous, or never autonomous person.

Early surgery does not clearly compromise later autonomy. However it may remove options that we believe should be available to people—that is, how their body is to appear. It may reduce important freedoms, but it does not clearly affect autonomy. Sharon Preves (1999) reports that although the in-depth life history interviews she carried out with intersex adults tell of "pain, sorrow, bewilderment, and anger," they also include accounts of "empowerment, identification, and reappropriation of intersexuality as a positive aspect of the self" (59). This capacity to cope with the stigma of being intersexed is suggestive of autonomy: "I don't think I would turn it in. I mean I've thought about this a lot. I really don't think that I would choose to be other than I am" (60). This comment reveals critical thinking and the ability to choose or change one's own attitude.

## CHILDREN'S DEVELOPING AUTONOMY

Although it does not make sense to talk about harm to the intersex child's future autonomy, it may make sense to talk about harm to a child's developing autonomy. Autonomy is not something that appears fully developed. Training children to become autonomous requires practice. Therefore, it might be claimed that aspects of the traditional medical model undermine or harm developing autonomy by not allowing the child to exercise choice or practice decision making. John Stuart Mill's (1948) argument about individuality as one of the elements of well-being could be interpreted as an argument about why we should value autonomy and why preventing children from making decisions can thwart the development of their autonomy (LaFollette 1998). Mill argues that we express our individuality and our humanity when we make choices.

Qualities such as "perception, judgement, discriminative feeling, mental activity, and even moral preference" are, according to Mill, the "distinctive endowment of a human being" and are exercised and developed only in the making of choices (51). The value is not in the choice but in Mill's idea of character or self-development (which we can interpret as autonomy) and in fully developing the necessary capacities:

> He who lets the world, or his own portion of it, choose his plan of life for him, has no need of any other faculty than the ape-like one of imitation. He who chooses his plan for himself, employs all his faculties. (51–52)

Some adult intersexuals tell of childhoods in which they lacked information about their conditions (a basic requirement for meaningful decision making) and lacked choice in the sense that they were not able to refuse repeated genital examinations performed without their consent:

> Because [the hospital I went to] is a teaching hospital, they would line up shoulder to shoulder all the way around from one side of the bed at the head, all the way across to the front and back up the other side. And everybody got a peek and a poke between my legs. And along about nine [years of age] that started getting real uncomfortable for me. But I was not allowed the power to say, "No, I don't want to play this game anymore." (Preves 2003, 66)

> You know while you're laying there that you don't have the right to say, "No. Stop. I don't want you to do this." (Preves 2003, 72)

How would such an experience undermine developing autonomy? The capacities needed for autonomy and making autonomous decisions need to be developed, and as mentioned previously, that requires practice. To some extent, it means we need to treat children as though they are already autonomous (LaFollette 1998). Preventing the exercise of choice may threaten developing autonomy, though it is not likely to undermine it entirely.

Helping intersexed children to develop autonomy is an important ethical consideration. But it is not clear that early surgery necessarily precludes that, as many opportunities for the exercise of choice in life still remain.

## DOES EARLY SURGERY MAKE AN
## INTERSEX INDIVIDUAL'S LIFE GO BETTER OR WORSE?

Though autonomy has been the main focus of ethical discussion, it is not the main ethical issue. The main ethical issue is the question, Does early surgery make the child's life go better or worse?

What is there about early surgery that can make the individual's life go worse?

- Poor surgical outcomes
- The attitude that intersexuality is shameful (Chase 1998, 385)

A poor surgical outcome is an obvious cause of harm, but it is not the only or the primary reason that former patients "feel harmed." Cheryl Chase (1998) argues that "the primary source of harm described by former patients is the underlying attitude that intersexuality is so shameful that it must be erased. . . . Early surgery is one means by which that message is conveyed to parents and to intersexed children." Another source of harm is the claim that "surgery is better now." This silences intersexed adults and "relieves surgeons indefinitely of the responsibility of listening to any former patient" (Chase 1998, 387).

The Intersex Society of North America (1998) refers to a "wealth of literature" expressing grief about the physical and emotional suffering caused by the surgery and anger toward the doctors who performed the surgery and the parents who consented to it. The society also places significance on the fact that there are no adults coming forward to say that they are grateful for having had early surgery performed.

The availability of literature about harm to intersex individuals who had early surgery is cause for concern, but it is not necessarily an indication that surgery made most intersex individuals lives go worse. It is possible that there is no audience for tales of successful surgery. Individuals who had surgery and are happy with it may not want to reveal their experience. What is more, unhappy outcomes would seem to be easier to name and describe, for example, in terms of grief and anger. How would we know if surgery made an individual's life go better? There is a need for information about the experience of those who feel that surgery was the right decision.

## PARENTAL ATTITUDES

There is some suggestion that parental attitude, rather than the decision to operate or not, has more influence on intersex children's successful development. In a study of children born with a small penis, "parental attitude" was reported to be the "strongest influence" on childhood experiences (Reilly and Woodhouse 1989). This study found that parents who were well informed and open with their children produced children who were "confident and well adjusted." Parents who were not open with their children, who focused on their abnormalities and told the child "to hide himself" produced shy, anxious, poorly adjusted children.

The importance of parental attitude is demonstrated further in the case of Ilizane Broks, a self-assured, seemingly well-adjusted 17-year-old with an intersex condition who has been brought up with full knowledge of her condition and "imbued" with a "healthy sense" of her "own identity and worth." She has been taught to "ignore the prejudice of the ignorant" and to be proud of her difference (Craig 2004). Ilizane has complete androgen insensitivity syndrome. She has both male and female genitalia. She looks like a girl, has a vagina but no uterus or ovaries, and has testes and XY chromosomes, which denote a boy. Ilizane overturns the image of the ostracized, cruelly teased intersex child. She delights in her father's story about her first day at school when she was a five-year-old. When each child was asked to stand on a chair and introduce themselves to the class, Ilizane climbed onto a chair and said: "Hello, my name is Ilizane. I'm not a girl and I'm not a boy . . . I'm an intersex!" Ilizane retains her early confidence, claiming she would like to be an actress: "I really like the idea of standing up in front of people and saying, 'Hey, this is me. Or rather, this isn't me. All is not as it seems.'"

In Ilizane's case, her parents resisted the suggestion to remove her testes and have left the decision to their daughter. Ilizane admits, however, that if she had congenital adrenal hyperplasia, the more common condition, she might have opted for surgery by now. The point being made here is that the child's environment matters—not in the sense that environment determines gender—but in the sense that acceptance and openness regarding the child's condition influences how well or how badly the child's life will go.

## KEY POINTS IN THE MANAGEMENT DECISIONS ABOUT INTERSEX

The preceding discussion suggests a number of points to bear in mind in minimizing harm:

- Surgery is most justified when there is a clear health risk.
- An early decision to do surgery (when appropriate) does not have to be a quick or rushed decision.
- One can assign a gender without doing surgery to match.
- Promote the idea that parental attitude is important. Parents who are informed and open tend to produce confident well-adjusted children (Reilly and Woodhouse 1989).
- Rather than promoting surgery or a moratorium on surgery, we should promote the idea that education, information, and positive attitudes in relation to intersex conditions matter most.
- It is important to look at the reason why a significant minority are not happy with the management of their condition.

It is still not clear what we should or should not do. Sometimes surgery has caused harm. Sometimes surgery may be the right decision. We need criteria to guide decisions.

A decision whether or not to perform surgery has to be made. In addition to the relevant medical facts, we need criteria to guide decisions on behalf of intersex newborns. Deference to parents as the most suitable people to be making medical decisions on behalf of their children (with help from doctors and with the relevant information) is based on the belief that parents are the best placed and most likely people to seek the best interests of their children. Nevertheless, given the controversy about early surgery for intersex newborns, the idea that parents should (1) leave the decision until the child is old enough to decide or (2) try to decide as the child would decide when old enough may seem like attractive options. But there are difficulties. First, leaving the decision for the child to decide when old enough carries the possibility of harm. It amounts to a decision not to perform early surgery rather than a way to respect autonomy. Second, in trying to decide as the child would, parents may end up making a decision that they *think* is not in their child's best interests—and that turns out *is not* in the child's best interests—based on an assumption about what a child who has not attained competence would decide when older (Dworkin 1988). Getting it wrong would surely be worse when parents make a decision that they do not believe in.

## CONCLUSION

The management of children born with intersex conditions raises many profound ethical issues, including those highlighted in box 4-3. It is often

---

**Box 4-3.  Why Management of Intersex Is an Important Ethical Issue**

The controversy surrounding the surgical management of intersex conditions in newborns is an important ethical issue because it:

- raises questions about the authority of parents and others to make irrevocable decisions for young children
- tests the idea that surgery is justified only when it is for disease or malfunction
- raises questions about what constitutes disease or malfunction
- questions the legitimacy of medical interventions that are carried out on one person in the interests of another
- helps shed light on the soundness of claims about threats to a child's future autonomy
- poses questions about what we should base treatment decisions on when there is little guidance in terms of evidence of outcomes
- illustrates the shift from physician-centered medicine and paternalism to patient-centered medicine and the need to listen to patient experience (narrative)
- highlights the need for evidence in the form of systematic outcomes studies

argued that the main ethical issue is about future autonomy. We have argued that freedom, but not future autonomy, may be compromised by early surgery to assign sex. It is important to promote the development of autonomy in children with intersex conditions, but this can be done in a number of ways, particularly including open disclosure of their condition and its management, without precluding early surgery. We have argued that the critical ethical issue is whether early surgery benefits or harms a particular individual in the sense of making that person's overall life go better or worse. Strikingly, there is very little empirical evidence to answer this question. The management of intersex speaks to the moral imperative to conduct ethically informed scientific research. Only then will we know what we should do.

## NOTES

This paper benefited from discussions with Garry Warne, Mary Rillstone, and other members of the Murdoch Childrens Research Institute Sex Study Group (MCRISSG).

1. It is difficult to interpret this case, as this individual had a twin brother whose death from an overdose of medication was a suspected suicide. See Chalmers 2004 and *CBC News* 2004.

2. *Secretary, Department of Health and Community Services* v. *J.W.B. and S.M.B.* ("Marion's Case") [1992] HCA 15; (1992) 175 CLR 218 F.C. 92/010 (6 May 1992). Marion's case involved an application for the sterilization of a 14-year-old teenager with a severe intellectual disability for the purpose of "preventing pregnancy and menstruation with its psychological and behavioural consequences."

3. Sentencia SU-337/99, May 12, 1999, and T-551/00, Aug. 2, 1999; quoted in Greenberg 2003, 279.

4. National Guideline Clearinghouse, available at www.guideline.gov.

5. Studies supporting early corrective genital surgery include Warne et al. 2005; Meyer-Bahlburg et al. 2004; and Migeon, Wisniewski, Gearhart et al. 2002; Migeon, Wisniewski, Brown et al. 2002. Studies which do not support early surgery include Minto et al. 2003; Creighton, Minto, and Steele 2001; May, Boyle, and Grant 1996; Dittman, Kappes, and Kappes 1992; and Reilly and Woodhouse 1989.

## REFERENCES

Aaronson, I. 2004. Editorial. *Journal of Urology* 171: 1619.

American Academy of Pediatrics, Committee on Genetics. 2000. Evaluation of the newborn with developmental anomalies of the external genitalia. *Pediatrics* 106 (1): 138–42.

Blackless, M., A. Charuvastra, A. Derryck, A. Fausto-Sterling, K. Lauzanne, and E. Lee. 2000. How sexually dimorphic are we? Review and synthesis. *American Journal of Human Biology* 12: 151–66.

Bullough, V. L. 2003. The contributions of John Money: A personal view. *Journal of Sex Research* 40 (3): 230–36.

*CBC News.* 2004. David Reimer: The boy who lived as a girl. *CBC News Online.* http://www.cbc.ca/news/background/reimer. May 10.

Chalmers, K. 2004. Sad end to boy/girl life: Subject of gender experiment. *Winnipeg Sun.* May 10. Available at http://www.canoe.ca/NewsStand/WinnipegSun/News/2004/05/10/453481.html.

Chase, C. 1998. Surgical progress is not the answer to intersexuality. *Journal of Clinical Ethics* 9 (4): 385–92.

Cohen-Kettenis, P. T., and F. Pfäfflin. 2003. *Transgenderism and intersexuality in childhood and adolescence: Making choices*. Vol. 46 of *Developmental clinical psychology and psychiatry*. Thousand Oaks, CA: Sage.

Craig, O. 2004. We are not what we seem. *Sunday Age*. Agenda section. March 28.

Creighton, S. M., C. L. Minto, and S. J. Steele. 2001. Objective cosmetic and anatomical outcomes at adolescence of feminising surgery for ambiguous genitalia done in childhood. *Lancet* 358 (9276): 124–25.

Daaboul, J., and J. Frader. 2001. Ethics and the management of the patient with intersex: A middle way. *Journal of Pediatric Endocrinology & Metabolism* 14: 1575–83.

Dittman, R. W., M. E. Kappes, and M. H. Kappes. 1992. Sexual behaviour in adolescent and adult females with congenital adrenal hyperplasia. *Psychoneuroendocrinology* 117 (2/3): 153–70.

Dreger, A. D., ed. 1999. *Intersex in the age of ethics*. Hagerstown, MD: University Publishing Group.

Dworkin, G. 1988. *The theory and practice of autonomy*. Cambridge: Cambridge University Press.

Eugster, E. A. 2004. Reality vs recommendations in the care of infants with intersex conditions—invited critique. *Archives of Pediatric and Adolescent Medicine* 158: 428–29.

Family Court of Australia. 1998. A question of right treatment: The Family Court and special medical procedures for children—An introductory guide for use in Victoria. Available at http://www.familycourt.gov.au/papers/pdf/vicmedical.pdf.

Feinberg, J. 1980. The child's right to an open future. In *Whose Child? Children's rights, parental authority, and state power*, ed. W. Aiken and H. LaFollette, 124–53. Totowa, NJ: Rowman & Littlefield. Reprinted in Joel Feinberg, *Freedom and fulfillment*, 76–97. Princeton, NJ: Princeton University Press, 1992.

Frader, J., P. Alderson, A. Asch, C. Aspinall, D. Davis, A. Dreger, J. Edwards, E. K. Feder, A. F., L. A. Hedley, E. Kittay, J. Marsh, P. S. Miller, W. Mouradian, H. Nelson, and E. Parens. 2004. Health care professionals and intersex conditions. *Archives of Pediatric and Adolescent Medicine* 158: 426–28.

Greenberg, J. 2003. Legal aspect of gender assignment. *Endocrinologist* 13 (3): 277–86.

Greenberg, J. A., and C. Chase. N.d. Background of Colombia decisions. Available at http://www.isna.org/drupal/book/view/21 (accessed September 7, 2004).

Intersex Society of North America. 1998. ISNA's amicus brief on intersex genital surgery. Available at http://www.isna.org/node/97.

Kipnis, K., and M. Diamond. 1998. Pediatric ethics and the surgical assignment of sex. *Journal of Clinical Ethics* 9 (4). Reprinted in Dreger 1999, 173–93.

LaFollette, H. 1998. Circumscribed autonomy: Children, care, and custody. In *Having and raising children*, ed. Uma Narayan and Julia J. Bartkowiak, 137–52. University Park: Pennsylvania State University Press.

Lawson Wilkins Pediatric Endocrine Society and European Society for Paediatric Endocrinology. 2002. Joint consensus statement on 21-hydroxylase deficiency from the Lawson Wilkins Pediatric Endocrine Society and the European Society for Paediatric Endocrinology. *J. Clin Endocrinol Metab* 87 (9): 4048–53.

Low, Y., J. Hutson, and Murdoch Childrens Research Institute Sex Study Group. 2003. Rules for clinical diagnosis in babies with ambiguous genitalia. *J. Paediatr. Child Health* 39 (6): 406–13.

May, B., M. Boyle, and D. Grant. 1996. A comparative study of sexual experiences. *Journal of Health Psychology* 1 (4): 479–92.

Mazur, T. 2004. A lovemap of a different sort from John Money: *A first person history of pediatric psychoendocrinology*—book review. *Journal of Sex Research* 41 (1): 115–16.

Meyer-Bahlburg, H., C. Migeon, G. Berkovitz, J. Gearhart, C. Dolezal, and A. Wisniewski. 2004. Attitudes of adult 46,XY intersex persons to clinical management policies. *Journal of Urology* 171: 1615–19.

Migeon, C. J., A. B. Wisniewski, T. R. Brown, John A. Rock, Heino F. L. Meyer-Bahlburg, John Money, and Gary D. Berkovitz. 2002. 46,XY intersex individuals: Phenotype and etiologic classification, knowledge of condition, and satisfaction with knowledge in adulthood. *Pediatrics* 110 (3): 32.

Migeon, C. J., A. B. Wisniewski, J. P. Gearhart, H. F. L. Meyer-Bahlburg, J. A. Rock, T. R. Brown, S. J. Casella, A. Maret, K. M. Ngai, J. Money, and G. D. Berkovitz. 2002. Ambiguous genitalia with perineoscrotal hypospadias in 46,XY individuals: Long-term medical, surgical, and psychosexual outcome. *Pediatrics* 110: 616–21.

Mill, J. S. 1948. On liberty. In *"On Liberty" and "Considerations on Representative Government,"* ed. R. B. McCallum, 1–104. Oxford: Basil Blackwell.

Minto, C. L., L.-M. Liao, C. R. J. Woodhouse, P. G. Ransley, and S. M. Creighton. 2003. The effect of clitoral surgery on sexual outcome in individuals who have intersex conditions with ambiguous genitalia: A cross-sectional study. *Lancet* 361: 1252–57.

Morris, E. 2004. The self I will never know. *New Internationalist* 364: 25–27.

Paediatric Surgeons Working Party. 2001. Statement of the British Association of Paediatric Surgeons Working Party on the Surgical Management of Children Born with Ambiguous Genitalia. Available at http://www.baps.org.uk/documents/Intersex%20statement.htm.

Preves, S. E. 1999. For the sake of the children: Destigmatizing intersexuality. In Dreger 1999, 50–65.

———. 2003. *Intersex and identity: The contested self.* New Brunswick: Rutgers University Press.

Purves, B. S. 2000. Parental consent and the surgical management of intersexed newborns. *Monash Bioethics Review* 9 (1): 23–42.

Rangecroft, L., on behalf of the British Association of Paediatric Surgeons Working Party on the Surgical Management of Children Born with Ambiguous Genitalia. 2003. Surgical management of ambiguous genitalia. *Arch Dis Child* 88: 799–801.

Reilly, J. M., and C. R. J. Woodhouse. 1989. Small penis and male sexual role. *Journal of Urology* 142: 569–71.

Reiner, W. G. 2004. Mixed-method research for child outcomes in intersex conditions. *BJU International* 93, suppl. (3): 51–53.

Sax, L. 2002. How common is intersex? A response to Anne Fausto-Sterling. *Journal of Sex Research* 39 (3): 174–78.

Schober, J. M. 2004. Feminizing genitoplasty: A synopsis of issues relating to genital surgery in intersex individuals. *Journal of Pediatric Endocrinology & Metabolism* 17: 697–703.

Spriggs, M. 1998. Autonomy in the face of a devastating diagnosis. *Journal of Medical Ethics* 24 (2): 123–26.

———. 2005. *Autonomy and patients' decisions.* Lanham, MD: Lexington Books.

Warne, G. Ethical issues in gender assignment. 2003. *Endocrinologist* 13 (3): 182–86.

Warne, G. L., S. Grover, J. Hutson, A. H. Sinclair, S. Metcalfe, E. Northam, J. Freeman, E. Loughlin, M. Rillstone, P. Anderson, E. Hughes, J. Hooper, S. Todd, J. D. Zajac, and J. Savulescu. 2005. A long-term outcome study of intersex conditions. *Journal of Pediatric Endocrinology & Metabolism* 18 (6): 555–67.

# 5

# Transsexualism and Gender Reassignment Surgery

*Heather Draper and Neil Evans*

The term *transsexual* is applied to people whose "gender identity is incongruent with their anatomical sex" (Herman-Jeglinska 2002, 527), that is, they believe themselves to be trapped in a body that is of the opposite sex to the one they believe themselves to be.[1] Gender reassignment surgery (GReS)[2] in conjunction with hormone therapy—particularly for male-to-female (MF) transsexuals—has been the treatment of choice (for both individuals and their doctors) for many decades now. Transsexualism has been recognized as a psychiatric classification (DSM IV [1994] 302.85) since 1980. The surgery is obviously very radical: genitalia are removed and replaced with reconstructed genitalia, breasts are removed or implants given, and vocal chords, along with teeth, noses, lips, and so forth may be altered to align them with the appearance of the desired sex. The surgical process is generally—but not always—spread over a series of months, and the hormone therapy will continue for life.

Clearly, such radical—some might say mutilating—surgery would be difficult to justify, even with the consent of the patient, without certainty about the following: that the patient's assertion is real rather than delusional (or put another way, that transsexualism is a genuine condition); that the therapy is effective; that the therapy is the only means of resolving the patient's problems; and, finally that the correct diagnosis has been reached. After all, healthy, functioning organs are removed and replaced by largely dysfunctional ones, and loss of spontaneous reproductive capacity is also inevitable.[3] Yet there remains controversy about whether transsexualism is a genuine condition, and there can therefore be no certainty that this is the best way of resolving the patient's problem. There is no compelling evidence about the effectiveness of the therapy of choice; and mistakes in diagnosis—assuming the possibility of correct diagnosis—are made with disastrous consequences for those who wrongly receive the surgery (Batty 2004). Yet around 5,000 GReSs have already been performed in the United Kingdom and the leading U.K. clinic plans to perform around 150 more of these in 2005 at a cost of at least £3000 each (Batty 2004), though the total cost facing a health authority is likely to be considerably more than this.[4]

Ethical debate about transsexualism was reignited in Australia in 2004 when the Family Court of Australia gave permission for a 13-year-old girl to begin hormone therapy as a prelude to possible reassignment surgery when she reached the age of majority.[5] Some of the debate seems to have been caused by a misunderstanding of the effects of the treatment, namely, that it was thought to have included the surgery itself or to be permanent in nature—which was not the case. Nonetheless, the concern of many commentators centered on whether it was right to give treatment to a minor for a condition of uncertain validity. Although it is arguably permissible not to interfere with an adult's decision to do something that seems grossly harmful from another's point of view, it seems even more contestable to facilitate the same process in a minor. Spriggs (2004) noted, however, that the court decision "was not about giving in to the unstable preferences of an immature person," but was rather about determining how best to accommodate her development needs.

It is interesting to note that our reactions to issues tangentially related to the question of whether transsexualism is an actual medical disorder illustrate how important it is to decide this issue. For instance, objections to transsexuals taking part in competitive sports, or to becoming fellows of the all-woman Newnham College at Cambridge University, or to having their birth certificates or passports reissued, all come back to the issue of whether such women or men are really what they claim to be or are only ever surgically reconstructed versions of their original selves.

In this chapter we will explore some of the reasons GReS is contested surgery and offer some suggestions for how, given these constraints, the surgery should be conducted.

## THE CASE OF
## SAM HASHIMI/SAMANTHA KANE/CHARLES KANE

The case of Sam Hashimi gained wide publicity in the United Kingdom during 2004, largely as a result of his own dealings with the media. Hashimi came to the United Kingdom as a student when he was 17. His first brush with publicity was in 1990 when, as a wealthy property developer, he made an unsuccessful takeover bid for a Sheffield football club. It is unclear from his various and inconsistent accounts whether he wrongly considered himself to be a transsexual as a result of losing his money, wife, and family or whether he always knew he was a transsexual. What is known is that Sam Hashimi became Samantha Kane during 1997.

As Samantha, Kane (1998) wrote a book about her experiences as an MF transsexual and, according to a subsequent documentary[6] also regained her wealth, though not her children's affections. Between 2003 and 2004 she was on a list of 12 patients whom colleagues of leading gender reassignment specialist Russell Reid claimed had been wrongly diagnosed and operated on. Reid was referred to the General Medical Council by these colleagues, and Kane made it known that she intended to sue Russell. The BBC documentary about Kane concerned his experiences as a wrongly diagnosed transsexual, which included following him through some of his therapies to be changed back to a man—Charles Kane.

Kane's case is unusual to the extent that Kane has been prepared to be a more public figure.[7] There are other reported instances, particularly of MF transsexuals seeking to get their surgery reversed.[8] The number of MF transsexuals seeking reversal is still only a small minority of all cases. The prevalence of MF requests for reversal probably reflects the fact that there appears to be somewhere between four and eight times more MF transsexuals than FM (female-to-male) ones (Raymond 1979, 24).

It is important to be sure about what such cases actually show. On the one hand, they have been used by critics of the whole notion of transsexualism to support the claim that it is a condition created by psychiatrists. On the other, all they may show is that doctors need to be extremely cautious in making a diagnosis and adhering to accepted guidelines before agreeing to perform surgery. For those concerned, undertaking surgery has left them suspended in a tragic limbo between male and female. It would be foolhardy in the extreme to assume that mistakes in diagnosis never occur, even in areas of medicine where there is absolutely no controversy about the condition misdiagnosed. However, when scalpels for hire undertake GReS, on the basis of only a short interview or basic physical appearance, it is unsurprising that mistakes—by both doctor and patient—are made.

Adhering to the strict guidelines, however, might not be acceptable to some transsexuals. Standard practice is for transsexuals to have at least three months of psychotherapy before beginning hormone therapy, and then to live as a member of their proclaimed sex for at least one year, full time and publicly—before undergoing any surgery (Harry Benjamin International Gender Dysphoria Association 2001). Given that transsexuals may wait for several years or even decades before presenting for help, a further wait can be frustrating. From the clinician's point of view, given that all there is to go on is the patient's sincere belief and ability to convince, the waiting period is an opportunity to be convinced over time, particularly when for a substantial period of this time the patient must experience the possible challenge to his/her beliefs of going public and facing the consequences in terms of negotiating new relationships with family, friends, and work colleagues. The waiting period is, then, also a test of resolve. However, from the point of view of the transsexual, particularly given that biomedical ethics and patient expectations are driven by patient autonomy and rights, this period can be viewed as unacceptably paternalistic. Let's return to the Kane documentary for a moment.

In this documentary, Kane is followed as he rather impulsively buys a boat. As the documentary continues, it becomes clear that Kane has no experience with boats (including how to navigate one as well as basic knowledge like how to start the engines). He is impatient with the bureaucracy surrounding boat sales and eventually begins to realize that he may not have bought the right boat, though he retains his image of himself with the boat that motivated the purchase. Our point here is that he was free to purchase this rather costly boat, and no one would dream of considering anyone negligent in having sold it to him. Even if we speculate that the agent "saw him coming" and was a tad unscrupulous in not ensuring that the boat fitted his needs, it would be difficult to argue that the agent had a duty not to sell the boat, or even to probe too deeply into what Kane needed most. Indeed, Kane might have been justifiably annoyed as a consumer having his judgment questioned if he was unwilling to seek advice in the first place. So, given that transsexuals themselves have a clear idea of what they want—even Kane, we must suppose, or else we would have also to question his current change of heart and subsequent surgery—then how can the waiting period be justified, especially when the patient is willing and perfectly able to pay for the surgery he or she wants?

The answer to this problem could be thought to lie in the difference between medicine and boat selling. Doctors have duties because health is of fundamental importance. Medicine, it has been claimed, is more than the mere gratification of a patient's preferences or the granting to patients of what makes them happy (Kass 1981). It is objective to the extent that the "state of an organism is theoretically healthy, i.e. free from disease, insofar as its mode of functioning conforms to the natural design of that kind of organism" (Boorse 1991, 57). Thus, the doctors' duty is based not just on the importance of promoting or restoring health but also on a shared understanding of what health is. And this returns us to the issue of whether transsexualism is a legitimate concern for medicine, and by implication a genuinely medical problem.

## THE EXTENT TO WHICH TRANSSEXUALISM IS A MEDICAL/SURGICAL PROBLEM

In the treatment of transsexualism, there is a convergence of three very different medical specialties: psychiatry, medicine, and surgery. The initial assessment, supervision, and monitoring falls to the psychiatrist; the patient is then referred to an endocrinologist, who takes responsibility for hormone and other therapies while a surgeon performs bodily reconstruction. This cooperation of specialties would appear to endorse the place of transsexualism within a medical model of disease or illness, but in each case there is a considerable divergence from normal practice in order to incorporate an ontological acceptance of transsexualism. We will focus particularly on psychiatry and surgery.

It is not unusual for psychiatrists to treat people who make claims that apparently challenge reality. For instance, in anorexia they would work on a woman's perception of herself as fat and try to realign her view of herself with the reality of her extreme thinness. Where transsexualism is unusual in psychiatry is that it is up to the patient to convince the psychiatrist that her view of herself, despite the "reality" of her body, is the correct one.[9] Thus, unlike the person with anorexia, the transsexual does not deny the facts of her male body: she is not trying to assert that her male penis is in fact a clitoris. Instead, she is arguing that it *ought* to be a clitoris. The transsexual's claim is based on some inner and unseen self that contradicts the facts about the external self. If there is a delusion operating here, then it is not a delusion about external appearances but about an inner self. In this respect, transsexualism is more like body dysmorphia.

In simple terms, then, in transsexualism the psychiatrist seeks to be convinced by the patient's view of reality, rather than the patient being convinced by the psychiatrist's, and it is only possible for the psychiatrist to be convinced if he has subscribed to the view that there *is* such a thing as transsexualism. Thus, the convincing that needs to be done centers around the sincerity and/or strength of the patient's own conviction, as measured against the psychiatrist's experience (either at first or second hand) with other transsexuals and their psychiatric histories. One aspect of this is the extent to which the patient is suffering as a result of her condition, which may take the form of suicidal tendencies, extreme unhappiness, and being unable to function socially (work, interact with family and friends, and so forth).

There are differing views about how transsexualism came to be accepted as a psychiatric condition. Hart and Wellings (2002) suggest that medical interest in the whole spectrum of human sexual behavior has its origins in the post-Victorian era where efforts were made to value the individual and his own suffering and to destigmatize certain individuals. Then there was the influence of the sexologists in particular, such as Havelock Ellis, who were part of medicine's general expansion into areas that had not traditionally been viewed as part of its remit. Out of such expansion medicine incorporated such human behaviors as masturbation, homosexuality, transvestism, and transsexuality. Finally, there was a general improvement in surgical techniques and discoveries in medicine (such as those related to hormones) that made treatment a possibility, though left the notion of transsexualism open to the same charge as other conditions that arose during the expansion of the medical boundaries, namely, that conditions of health or unhealthiness are related more to the possibility of "cure" than to concepts of health per se (infertility could be another example here).

From the point of view of psychiatry, however, another general criticism is that the treatments on offer alter the *body* when the condition itself seems to have its origins in the *mind*. Of course, much of modern psychiatric practice involves altering the body, primarily the brain, using chemicals. So perhaps the challenge should be rephrased: if, as some psychiatrists hypothesize, transsexualism is caused by some malfunction in the wiring in the brain during fetal development, and if drugs were developed that could make good this wiring, would the treatment of preference continue to be the realignment of the body with the beliefs of the individual, or would it be to realign the perception with the body? Restoring the wiring to working order would be to cure transsexualism, whereas GReS concentrates only on the symptoms and thus could be argued to produce surgically constructed men and women (Raymond 1979, xvi n 5); put even more strongly, GReS turns "men into fake women and women into fake men" (Szasz 1980, 86–87).

Ironically, to argue that, given the choice, we should opt to treat the brain, and therefore the perception of the transsexual, suggests that the perception of the transsexual is actually a false one, which in turn undermines not the sincerity of the transsexuals claim but the truth of the claim, and therefore the validity of GReS. This does not mean that performing GReS is wrong: it could still be argued to be a pragmatic response to extreme suffering using what is currently available. So the current situation could be characterized in terms of what we can do technically determining treatment, which in turn determines diagnosis. If we accept that what is currently happening is a pragmatic approach, rather than one that accepts the truth of what is claimed, it makes sense for psychiatrists to base a referral for radical surgery on proof of the extreme unhappiness of the patient and evidence that they are sincere in the beliefs about their gender and steadfast in their resolve to seek surgery. The extreme unhappiness might justify surgery within the current model of medical ethics, where no intervention should be given unless the harms outweigh the benefits. Thus surgery can be considered worthwhile on balance, even if the condition does not actually exist in quite the way that the transsexual believes.

Turning to surgery, this same on-balance justification could be employed, even though it could be contested when measured against the normal practice of surgery. Normally a surgeon would expect to remove or repair only diseased tissue, organs, or limbs, yet this is not what is happening in GReS where healthy, but undesired, organs are removed. However, there are other departures from normal practice that still fit comfortably with the surgical model, for instance, surgical sterilization or removal of healthy tissue for transplantation into another person. The "fit" seems to depend both on the acceptability to the surgeon of the existence of the condition and how extreme it is. Thus, removal of a healthy kidney for transplantation purposes is acceptable, but removal of a healthy heart would not be; likewise, GReS seems to be acceptable, while, in the United Kingdom at least, few surgeons would be comfortable removing two or more limbs in the case of body dysmorphia.

We have already looked at the question of how plausible the whole notion of transsexualism is, and clearly any surgeon performing the surgery must be prepared either to accept that transsexualism is a genuine condition or accept the "on balance justified" argument. But there are a series of other interrelated issues that arise for the surgeon. The first is how effective surgery is likely to be, since if it is not very effective this would affect the "on balance" judgment. Next is the question of whether the results have to be plausible—whether, for instance, the MF transsexual will pass readily as a woman. Finally there is the question of whether the surgery should be aimed solely at reconstruction or if it is necessary for the surgeon to create for the transsexual the woman or man he/she desires to become—the "ideal" or "perfect" man or woman.

There are two senses in which GReS can be judged to be effective or not: there is technical success, judged totally in terms of the surgical procedures, and success in terms of whether the patient feels better or more balanced as a result of having their gender reassigned. While the latter is in part dependant on the former, what is important from the point of view of the justification for performing the surgery is the latter: the surgery could be a success locally but fail in terms of the global project of improving the patient's quality of life. There is conflicting evidence of success taken globally. While there are papers purporting to have illustrated success, the Aggressive Research Intelligence Facility (ARIF) of the University of Birmingham, England, does not consider that the issue of effectiveness can be settled on the basis of the evidence currently available.[10] Moreover, there is much less evidence relating to FM transsexuals than to MF transsexuals. This is in part due to the smaller numbers but could also be due to a reluctance of FM transsexuals to draw any kind of attention to themselves (Raymond 1979, xxii). Lack of *conclusive* evidence of effectiveness does not, however, mean that it is not effective—especially as, in the current economic climate, it is not sufficient to show that an intervention is effective; it must also be *more* effective than other interventions in a randomized control trial. As ARIF observes, a trial aiming to randomize transsexuals in trial arms that would include psychotherapy only or doing nothing only as well as GReS are unlikely to recruit sufficient, if any, participants.

What we do know from retrospective research is that two factors seem to point to greater overall success. The first of these is the age at which surgery is performed (Lawrence 2003, 300) and the age at onset of the feelings of being a transsexual. The older one is, in each case, the less likely one is to be satisfied postsurgery. The second is the extent to which the surgery is unproblematic or successful in its own right. This brings in the two further related issues mentioned above: plausibility and conformity to desires.

The job of the surgeon here is to reassign gender, but for gender reassignment to be successful, it must also be plausible. The MF should be able to pass as a woman and the FM as a man, one aspect of which is being able to be attract sexual attention[11] from genetic men/women rather than reconstructed men/women, irrespective of sexual orientation. This might depend on physical characteristics that are not very amenable to surgical correction such as height and build. If the success of the surgery is based at least in part on how plausible the results are likely to be, then plausibility is likely, consciously or unconsciously, to become one criterion in the assessment of the suitability of transsexuals for GReS. This may, however, undermine other aspects of the assessment, such as testing the sincerity of the patient's belief or the resolve to continue.[12]

Plausibility is, however, quite a different goal from the one that the transsexual might set for him/herself. Many transsexuals seek not just to change sex but to end up as a conventionally attractive member of the opposite sex. The desire to be physically attractive is common, but in terms of GReS what might otherwise be classed as a cosmetic effect appears more fundamental. So, for instance, a typical MF transsexual is likely to want to be and appear to be more feminine than an average genetic woman (Herman-Jeglinska 2002). Bound up with the conviction that he is truly female may be the desire to be an attractive female conforming to cultural norms of female beauty such as prettiness, thinness, femininity, desirability to the opposite sex, demureness, and provocativeness. For the transsexual, this means that cosmetic surgery might not be viewed as an optional extra to the GReS but part and parcel of changing gender. This can lead to differing expectations of what counts as success between the patients and their surgeons.

The surgeons could be defended for arguing that their role is to reassign sex, and so while they might not oppose cosmetic surgery in principle, they might argue that requests for what they perceive as cosmetic surgery should be judged alongside other (i.e., nontranssexual) patients' requests for enhancement and perhaps would not be available using public funds. Perhaps, then, all the surgeon contracts to do is to make a constructed woman/man rather than an *attractive* constructed woman/man.

This is important when considering how well a surgeon can be said to have done her job, or in a worst-case scenario, whether she can be considered negligent or to have in some other way failed her patient. Thus there might be two standards against which the surgery can be judged: the objective assessment of whether the surgery was carried out with due care (for example, avoiding unnecessary scarring, employing modern techniques competently, and so on), and the subjective judgment of the patient about whether the surgery has made her the kind of woman she wanted to be as opposed to simply making her a woman. We would argue that it is in the former that the duty of the surgeon lies, but this is not straightforward.

A transsexual person can be thought of, along with all others, as existing through three dimensions of the self: past, present, and future. The past self for the transsexual is the suffering self, the self that existed from earliest times as an isolated, estranged, unhappy, and dispossessed misfit. This past self often contemplated suicide and eventually sought medical help to alleviate the distress. The present self (now diagnosed as a transsexual) is a self on a journey, a transitional self moving forward. Nothing for this person is permanent because everything else in life is on hold, awaiting surgery. It is the future self exclusively that matters. It is the female self that is achieved following surgery that is the self that will know fulfillment, happiness, and recognition. This future self is to be revealed when all the surgical bandages are removed and she stands in front of a mirror for herself and all others to see. This is the moment of realization and of completion. This is the moment that life will begin for the first time and unhappiness will become a thing of the past.

In her autobiography *Conundrum*, Jan Morris writes of her response when she looked at herself in the mirror following surgery. Her physical appearance at last corresponded to the inner feelings that she had possessed for so long. In turn her new physicality impacted upon her inner experience in a way that was pleasing to her.

> It is not merely the loss of androgens that has made me more retiring, more ready to be led, more passive: the removal of the sex organs themselves has contributed; for there was to the presence of the penis something positive, thrusting and muscular. My body was then made to push and to initiate and it is now made to yield and accept and the outside change has had its inner consequences. (1974, 141)

This comment seems to demonstrate Morris's desire to conform to stereotypical views of femininity and the way in which surgery, especially as a result of the removal of the penis, accomplished this.

These divisions of the self are not absolute, as they coexist and overlap, but they provide a useful way of clarifying goals and concerns. To which self does the surgeon and psychiatrist owe a duty of care? Is it to the past suffering self—in which case, the motivation for performing GReS becomes one of alleviating and not creating further suffering? Or is it to the present self for whom surgery becomes a means or *the* means of achieving realization? Or is it to the future self—in which case, the surgeon may be agreeing to create a future self that brings about the dreams and wishes of the transsexual that include being sculpted into an attractive as well as plausible woman.

The pre-op transsexual has an unusually heavy investment in her future self. It could be argued that she is almost exclusively investing in her future self. Such investment is inherently problematic, though not only does it lead to a truncated appreciation of the present life but it also carries with it the increased possibility that such investment will fail to bring the hoped-for returns (as it does for anyone living primarily in the future). To exclusively focus upon a future self in the belief that realizing that self will be the equivalent of entering the Promised Land is first to nurture false beliefs and second to create a condition in which disillusionment is a real possibility.

Thus, from this perspective, the transsexual may feel that it is legitimate to hold the surgeon responsible for any failure to make her an attractive woman because it is the surgeon who is constructing her as a woman. A genetic woman may regard herself as unattractive but, adverse incidents aside, has no one to blame for this. It seems to us, then, vital that it be made clear to the transsexual from the outset that the purpose of the surgery is to reassign gender and not to make an ideal (according to the patient) woman.

## PROCEEDING WITH TREATMENT

What we have established so far is that although there could be grounds for suspecting that transsexualism is not a genuine condition in the sense that someone of one gender *is* trapped inside the body of the opposite gender, there are grounds for treating those that suffer as a result of their transsexual beliefs with GReS as a pragmatic response to an otherwise insoluble and debilitating condition. This justification is based on surgery being of benefit to the patient *on balance*. However, such a justification must require certain safeguards and precautions.

We have noted that in order to make a diagnosis, a psychiatrist has to be convinced of the sincerity of the transsexual's beliefs, and that in order to refer the patient for GReS, there must also be certainty about the resolve of the patient both to publicly live as a member of the opposite gender—with all the consequences that will flow for relationships with family, friends, and work colleagues—and to face repeated surgical procedures. It is clear from the Harry Benjamin guidelines that not all transsexuals require GReS; some are content with hormone therapy only, some do not even wish to live as a member of the opposite sex. Likewise, not all transsexuals want to undergo a complete gender reassignment: some FM transsexuals, while happy to live as a male, do not want to undergo penile construction but are content to go only as far as having breasts, ovaries, and uterus removed. So even though there is a sense in which, as we have explained, the possibility of GReS has facilitated the emergence of a diagnosis of transsexualism, this does not mean that GReS naturally follows from diagnosis. Thus, psychiatrists have an obligation to explore with the patient what is required for her to live a more balanced life. This is an unsurprising conclusion in the age of informed consent. However, if we also recall that the justification for surgery is an on-balance one, it is arguable that psychiatrists should be trying first and foremost to assess how *little* intervention is necessary to improve the patient's quality of life, rather than simply assessing whether they are informed about and prepared for the consequences of GReS.

Against this background and notwithstanding the arguments already outlined in relation to paternalism, the Harry Benjamin guidelines on both eligibility and readiness for GReS criteria are not just prudent in terms of defending negligence claims, but an ethical requirement. These require that the patient has reached the age of majority, has received hormone therapy for at least 12 months, has had 12 months successful *continuous* real-life experience (as opposed to real-life tests) of living as a member of the opposite sex, and has demonstrated progress in consolidating a gender identity and also that the continuous real-life experience has had an overall positive effect on his/her mental health. Although psychotherapy is not a requirement, given the criteria and the need for assessment, a therapeutic relationship of at least 12 months' standing seems to be built into the guidelines. Moreover, it seems to us that those seeking a reversal of GReS, too, should meet the same criteria. The Harry Benjamin guidelines also recommend long-term follow-up, though it is difficult to see how the psychiatrist can ensure the patient's cooperation with this.

One moot point is the extent to which the transsexual is obliged to take account the affects of her decision on her family members, particularly children who are still minors. Clearly, no self-respecting psychiatrist would fail to discuss these with her patient. But exploring how a patient will cope with and manage upheaval is different from asking whether the patient is entitled to visit such upheaval on others, especially minor children. What we are seeking to challenge here is one of the precepts of modern psychotherapy, namely, that everyone *deserves* to be happy. Of course, this is not just an issue for transsexual parents; it is also an issue for would-be separating parents or indeed all parents. It is difficult to judge what the balance ought to be between self-fulfillment and our obligations to our children. We do not have time here for an extensive consideration of the issues; we merely want to raise the possibility that transsexuals have obligations to others as well as themselves and to suggest that these obligations also warrant serious ethical, as opposed to psychiatric, consideration. This might commit a transsexual to never having GReS or it might be the case that GReS can be delayed, giving weight to the obligations of the existing person as well of those of the future person they would like to become. Those advocating publicly funded GReS must also be aware that as well as committing public funds to the immediate and long-term treatment of the transsexual person, they may also be committing funds to the immediate and long-term care of her family. Likewise, those who consider that GReS paid for by the patient herself raises fewer ethical concerns should consider whether the transsexual should also commit to fund the health care of any dependants affected by her decisions.

Returning to the actual surgery, what are the obligations of the surgeon? Surgeons are not merely technicians; if they want to remain members of the medical profession, they have to abide by professional standards, and this means being more than surgically competent. The treatment of transsexuals is a team effort involving psychiatrists, endocrinologists, and surgeons. The psychiatrist takes the lead role in the diagnosis and assessment of the patient, and it is not unreasonable for the surgeon and endocrinologist to depend upon the psychiatrist's judgment. But this should not be an uncritical trust. As professionals, they must also be satisfied both ontologically and in terms of individual patients that intervention is necessary. This means that they should not be treating any patients who are not under the care of a psychiatrist (one who has experience of transsexualism) and they should not treat any patient who has not fulfilled the Harry Benjamin criteria of eligibility and readiness. While the surgeon cannot also be expected to undertake a psychiatric assessment, she can be expected to satisfy herself that such an assessment has been made by at least one, if not two, suitably qualified psychiatrists.

Further than this, the surgeon also has an obligation to ensure that her expectations for the surgery are in line with those of the patient. Based on our previous discussion, and again in line with conventional thinking about consent, this may involve explicit discussion with the patient about what can be realistically achieved with GReS and possibly later with cosmetic surgery.

A surgeon performing GReS cannot be held responsible for not constructing an attractive male or female, only for not performing with due skill and competence, but such a surgeon could be held responsible for holding out false promise or for not ensuring that the patient has realistic expectations of what they will look like when the bandages are removed and the scars heal.

## NONMEDICAL ETHICS ISSUES

In this chapter, we have concentrated on GReS as a contested form of surgery in the context of medical ethics. To close, we would like to mention some aspects of transsexualism and GReS that we do not have time to explore in detail.

First, we have not explored the nature of gender and its social construction. Historically, gender was thought of as coexistent with the sex of the body and thus was essentially dimorphic. Male characteristics were assumed to belong to the male body and vice versa. However, as a result of the gradual medicalization of human sexual behavior (as discussed above), John Money (1955) was able to introduce a concept of gender that owed its origin to the linguistic nature of the term and served as a way of distinguishing between feminine and masculine *character* traits and those that are *biological*. Thus a way was open to construct notions of gender that were independent of bodily considerations. This in turn had consequences for medicine with regard to the legitimacy of transsexualism as a medical condition and for feminism in its attempts to eradicate sexual and gender dimorphism as an expression of masculine and paternalistic power dynamics. Without such a distinction between gender and sex, the concept of transsexualism would have been impossible.

Second, we tried to show how GReS is contestable from within a mainstream view of medical ethics. But there are other ways of exploring what the concept of transsexualism means, how we should respond to it and its implications for society. Janice Raymond (1979), for instance, writes about the implications for feminism of accepting the concept of MF transsexualism and GReS and welcoming what she terms "she-males" within feminism. In the preface to the *Transsexual Empire*, she warns:

> What goes unrecognised, consciously or unconsciously, by women who accept such transsexuals as women and as lesbian feminists is that their masculine behaviour is disguised by the castration of the male "member." Loss of a penis, however, does not mean the loss of an ability to penetrate women—women's identities, women's spirits, women's sexuality . . . the transsexually constructed lesbian-feminist not only colonizes female bodies but appropriates a feminist "soul." (xix)

Finally, we have not addressed the legal and social issues that greatly perplex postoperative transsexuals. Although some governments do have policies to ensure that transsexuals have equal rights in terms of access to health care resources, employment protection, and other social benefits,[13] there remain certain sticking points, particularly related to the changing of birth certificates and the right to marry. Concerns have also been raised about the extent to which transsexualism can be accommodated within sporting competitions as the combination of different sex and gender might give postoperative transsexual competitors an unfair advantage over genetic men or women.

## NOTES

This paper was a collaboration of equal effort. Our thanks go to Professor Femi Oyebode and other members of the Dept of Psychiatry, Birmingham University for helpful comments on a presentation on transsexualism given as part of the postgraduate education programme on Psychiatry in Birmingham.

1. The ICD-10 judged transsexualism according to three criteria: "1. The desire to live and be accepted as a member of the opposite sex, usually accompanied by the wish to make his or her body as congruent as possible with the preferred sex though surgery and hormone treatment; 2. The transsexual identity has been persistent for at least two years; 3. The disorder is not a symptom of another mental disorder or chromosomal abnormality" (Harry Benjamin International Gender Dysphoria Association 2001).

2. Sometimes also referred to as "sex reassignment surgery" or "sex-change operation."

3. Gametes can be stored, but it is difficult to see how useful they would be given that most transsexuals claim also to be heterosexual.

4. The Suffolk Health Authority (1994) estimated this to be in the region of £50,000 more than 10 years ago.

5. *Re Alex: hormonal treatment for gender identity dysphoria* [2004] FamCA 297.

6. BBC1, "Make Me a Man Again," October 19, 2004.

7. Charles Kane is now reported to be writing a new book, *Back on Mars from a Long Trip to Venus.*

8. See, for instance, Batty 2004.

9. The assumption here is not that all transsexuals are male to female; the designation of "she," etc., is used simply for reasons of style.

10. The available evidence reviewed and their reasons can be found online at http://www .arif.bham.ac.uk/Requests/g/genderreass.htm.

11. Which is not be the same thing as being generally sexually attractive, that is, conventionally beautiful or handsome.

12. Batty (2004) suggests that there is too much emphasis on plausibility in the history of those who consider that their surgery was a mistake.

13. For a summary of the British government policy, see http://www.dca.gov.uk/ constitution/transsex/policy.htm.

# REFERENCES

Batty, D. 2004. Mistaken identity. *Guardian*, July 31. Available at http://society.guardian.co.uk/ health/story/0,7890,1273045,00.html.

Boorse, C. 1991. On the distinction between disease and illness. In *Medicine and Moral Philosophy*, ed. M. Cohen, T. Nagel, and T. Scanlon. Princeton, NJ: Princeton University Press.

Harry Benjamin International Gender Dysphoria Association. 2001. Standards of care for gender identity disorders. 6th ed. Minneapolis: Harry Benjamin International Gender Dysphoria Association. Available at http://www.hbigda.org/soc.htm.

Hart, G., and K. Wellings. 2002. Sexual behaviour and its medicalisation. *British Medical Journal* 324: 896–900.

Herman-Jeglinska, A. et al. 2002. Masculinity, femininity, and transsexualism. *Archives of Sexual Behavior* 31 (6): 527–34.

Kane, S. 1998. *A two-tiered existence.* London: Writers and Artists.

Kass, L. 1981. Regarding the end of medicine and the pursuit of health. In *Concepts of health and disease: Interdisciplinary perspectives*, ed. A. Caplan, H. T. Engelhardt Jr., and J. J. McCartney. Reading, MA: Addison-Wesley.

Lawrence, A. 2003. Factors associated with satisfaction or regret following male–female sex reassignment surgery. *Archives of Sexual Behavior* 32 (4): 300.

Money, J. 1955. Linguistic resources and psychodynamic theory. *British Journal of Medical Psychology* 28: 264–66.

Morris, J. 1974. *Conundrum.* London: Faber & Faber.

Raymond, J. G. 1979. *The transsexual empire.* London: Women's Press.

Spriggs, M. P. 2004. Ethics and the proposed treatment of a 13-year-old with atypical gender identity. *Medical Journal of Australia* 181 (6): 319–21.

Suffolk Health Authority. 1994. Transsexuals and sex reassignment surgery. Internal report. Available at "Press for Change," http://www.pfc.org.uk/medical/suffolk.htm.

Szasz, T. 1980. *Sex: Facts, frauds and follies.* Oxford: Blackwell.

# III

# SEPARATING CONJOINED TWINS

# 6

## ✢

# Separating Conjoined Twins: Disability, Ontology, and Moral Status

## *Richard Hull and Stephen Wilkinson*

The contested surgery examined in this chapter is the separation of conjoined twins. In particular, we concern ourselves with two claims: one about the health status of conjunction, the other about the moral-ontological status of conjoined twins. The first says that being conjoined is a "mere difference" rather than a disorder, disability, or impairment—that conjunction is a difference, not a defect. The second says that conjoined twins have a moral and/or ontological status which is significantly different from that of other twins. We argue that both these claims are false, or at least that there are no compelling arguments for them. This does not have any direct implications for the question of whether separation is permissible. However, since both claims are sometimes used in antiseparation arguments, showing them to be implausible may, in some circumstances, reinforce the case for separation by weakening certain antiseparation assertions.

Many of the arguments discussed in this chapter are general insofar as they apply to all or most conjoined twins. However, in order to screen out a number of complications, particularly those relating to valid consent, we focus throughout (unless otherwise stated) on infant conjoined twins (Wilkinson 2003). We also focus on cases in which each twin has its own functioning brain since, as Bratton and Chetwynd (2004, 280) point out, the scenario in which one twin is "just some extra flesh attached . . . would present no ethical problems"—or at least no special ethical problems relating to conjunction.

## IS CONJUNCTION A DISABILITY?

In this section we argue that conjunction (being conjoined) is both a physical impairment and a disability. How significant that disability is, or need be, is a more complicated issue that will also be explored.

First, something needs to be said about disability in general. Many debates about disability assume that it is either a purely medical condition or a purely social problem. It has been argued at greater length elsewhere that it is generally "a bit of both" (Hull 1998). We should not overlook the fact of physical impairment or functional limitation when we are thinking about disability. Nor should we overlook the role of social structures, attitudes, and arrangements. The problem with the (purely) medical model of disability is that it ascribes too much weight to impairment. Disability is said to *result* from impairment in a way that suggests a direct and inevitable connection, but this is simply false in many cases. For example, inadequate welfare measures, education, health and social support services, housing, transport, and built environments do not simply and inevitably *result* from impairment, nor does institutional or personal discrimination. Yet these are the sorts of things that comprise much of the experience of disability for people with impairments. Rather obviously, they need not just follow or result from the fact of impairment; they depend on how a society responds, or fails to respond, to the needs of some of the people within that society. Thus, many disabilities would be much less disabling if society were differently organized. For example, if ramps and lifts were more common than stairs, people who rely on wheelchairs to get around would be much less disabled than they presently are.

Functional limitation necessitates disability only if the activity in question requires the use of the functionally limited part or system. So, for example, if I have a seriously defective right kneecap, then that on its own will prevent me from performing any activities involving running. If, however, declaring my defective kneecap in a job application (when the job involves no running whatsoever) prevents me from getting the job, because of the selectors' discriminatory attitudes toward people with defective kneecaps, that is an entirely different matter—and here the disability is dependent on social attitudes and structures. Of course, things are rarely this simple in reality. Disability more often than not involves a highly complex interplay of impairment and social factors. Nonetheless, it is useful to distinguish disabilities that result primarily from impairment from those that result primarily from a socially inadequate or discriminatory response to impairment, when we are thinking about disability issues and, specifically, about conjoined twins. Disability is not just a social phenomenon, but rarely is it a purely medical one either. Each conventional model captures one, but only one, aspect of disability.

Causes aside, disability tends to concern us because of the impact it can have on our capacity to flourish as human beings. As Glover argues:

> Disability requires failure of functioning. But failure of functioning creates disability only if (on its own or *via* social discrimination) it impairs capacities for human flourishing. It would not be a disability if there were a failure of a system whose only function was to keep toenails growing. With arrested toenail growth, we flourish no less. (2006, 5)

Thus, it is the impact that a particular functional limitation has, "either on its own or—more usually—in combination with social disadvantage" (Glover 2006, 6), on our capacity to flourish as human beings that is critical to the evaluation of how severe a particular disability is and, by implication, whether we should try to do something about it.[1] With respect to conjunction, then, we should ask both whether it amounts to a functional limitation and, if it does, what its likely impact on flourishing is.

In what follows, we attempt to strip away all incidentals and consider conjunction in a very simplified, and thus rather unrealistic, way. Conjunction often brings with it "serious physiological concerns," such as the inability to walk without aid (Dreger 2004, 53–56). However, for the purposes of inquiring as to whether conjunction is a functional limitation per se, we will leave aside any functional limitations that are often *associated with* conjunction. We will assume that, other than the presence of an anatomical bond, all other functioning is species typical.

Conjunction implies some sort of restriction of the use of the part of the body where the anatomical bond is located. One[2] will not be able to move that part of one's body freely and it is unlikely that one will be able to move freely, nor determine the movement of, that which one is joined to. That clearly denotes a functional difference and, inasmuch as one is unable to move as freely as one could without the anatomical bond, a functional limitation. Moreover, the implied need for cooperation from one's twin, while not functionally limiting per se, could entail that one is functionally limited by another. However, that may be to move away from what we traditionally see as functional limitation. It may be described better as potential noncooperation or an external functional limitation.

That aside, it is clear that the site of conjunction will be both functionally limited and functionally limiting, with the degree of restriction depending on the location and scale of the join. For example, the most common form of conjunction is *parapagus*, which entails that twins are "intimately joined at the pelvic region and sometimes also much farther up the body, toward the head." The site of conjunction is extensive and can include the joining of limbs; "it generally looks as if there are two persons at the upper end of the body and one at the lower end" (Dreger 2004, 29). In contrast, *omphalopagus* twins (joined at the umbilical region) can have a less extensive site of conjunction leaving all limbs free. Functional limitation will generally be less substantial in the latter case than the former.

Conjunction then inevitably involves *some* degree of physical impairment or functional limitation. So given this, what disadvantages or disabilities are likely to result? The most obvious is lack of privacy—or inability to be in a private space. The ability to be in a private space is something that we tend to take for granted, whether or not it is conditional to our flourishing (something explored below). For now, it is sufficient to note that, insofar as we value privacy and the modes of life and life choices associated with it, the inability to be in a private space will constitute an impediment to our capacity to flourish.

Closely related to lack of privacy is the inability to go anywhere or do very much without the cooperation of a third party.[3] There will be a need for compromise over major lifestyle issues: for example, both twins may not be able to pursue their preferred careers. And so conjunction is disabling insofar as independent choice and action are valuable, which often they are. Also, depending on the location and extent of the site of conjunction, there may be mobility disabilities related to, for example, loss of limb function. How serious these disabilities are will, again, depend on which activities are precluded by these functional limitations, and on the importance and value of these activities.

Leaving aside disabilities that can result from other serious physiological concerns often associated with conjunction, it will already be clear that the impact of a given disability is very much bound up with views about what counts as an acceptable or desirable form or aspect of human life. Judgments about this can be difficult and contentious. Moreover, they tend to be mediated by considerations about what is normal, which can also be controversial. However, that does not mean that we cannot, or should not, attempt to make them. Indeed, it is important that we do.

As Glover notes, the boundary between normality and disability is often a blurred one, "a continuum of severity." He adds, "We only count functional limitations as disabilities when there is a contrast with normal human functioning" (2006, 7). Some idea of normal or species-typical functioning is always at work; it is departures from the norm that can denote what we consider to be disabling (e.g., see Buchanan et al. 2000, 72). However, as Glover also notes, what we consider to be normal is within a social context that may not remain static. "If a widespread mutation (or widespread use of genetic engineering) gave most people wings, those of us unable to fly might start to count as disabled" (8). Moreover, in a similar way to that seen earlier with disability, what we consider to be normal might have a considerable social component. So, for example, if a majority with wings started to build public buildings without stairs, ramps, or lifts to *any* floors and started to build houses in the tops of trees, those without wings would face considerable dis-

advantages. Yet those disadvantages would have much more to do with social structures, attitudes, and arrangements than they would with the newly
defined imposition of being unable to fly. Thus, we should be acutely aware
of the social context of what we consider to be normal and, potentially, the
social influence upon that very definition.

However, "accepting that the boundaries of normal functioning may to
some extent be context-dependent and may have an element of social construction is consistent with seeing normal human functioning as providing
the background contrast to the limitations that count as contributing to disabilities" (Glover 2006, 8). Moreover, the background contrast is only important here insofar as it furnishes us with a deeper understanding of what is
likely to contribute to or detract from our flourishing as human beings. Being without wings in a high-flying society, for example, may not matter very
much at all, especially if that society remained *or became* sympathetic in all
respects to the flightless. Yet it could come to matter a lot, for a variety of reasons, and inasmuch as the contrast with normal functioning might explain
why, it is a useful point of comparison. Indeed, acknowledging the potential
difficulties with an account of normal human functioning should make it
more useful rather than less.

Having said that, the contrast with normal species functioning is only
one source of understanding. Another is actual accounts and preferences
of people living with a particular condition such as conjunction. With respect to independent choice and action, for example, Dreger writes that
"conjoinment does not automatically negate individual development and
expression, any more than other forms of profound human relations do.
Indeed, differing personalities and tastes are the rule among conjoined
twins with two conscious heads" (2004, 40). According to Dreger, "the evidence tells us that conjoined twins who have remained conjoined do in
fact become individuals in the psychological sense, if not in the physical
sense; each speaks of him- or herself as an individual, and they develop
personalities and tastes distinct from those of their siblings" (44). Moreover, "the notion that a conjoined twin must individuate to the same degree singletons do takes singleton development, unjustifiably, as the standard for everyone" (44).

Dreger suggests that conjunction does not significantly reduce flourishing,
citing as evidence the "practically universal" desire among communicating
conjoined twins to remain together:

> People who are conjoined and able to communicate seem to be almost as disin-
> clined to be surgically separated as singletons are to be surgically joined. The Bi-
> janis' remains the only case in which conjoined twins old enough to express
> preferences have consented to separation. Moreover, conscious conjoined peo-
> ple whose twins have died have invariably chosen to remain attached, knowing
> that this means that they will soon also die, and that in the interim they will be
> attached to their dead sibling. (2004, 46)

Dreger also provides an account of the positive aspects of being conjoined. She talks of conjoined twins being "never lonely" (34), "models of co-operative behaviour" (40), armed with a "double strength and a double will" (44), and describing their lives as "like being born with your soul mate" (49). Such considerations, according to Dreger, should "lead the thoughtful, sympathetic singleton to consider the degree to which any of us truly are or wish to be independent of others, and to ask why individuality—or any other aspect of humanity—need be thought of as limited to one particular kind of anatomy" (50). Indeed, she asks whether "we might not all benefit from more twin-type behaviour in this world—that is, whether we might not *all* benefit from a little *less* 'individuation'" (44).

Dreger's account rightly encourages critical reflection on some of the commonly made assumptions about conjoined twins. However, such reflection should not be at the expense of some crucial points. First, as Dreger (63) notes, the fact that conjoined twins almost invariably state that they are not trapped or confined by their conjunction raises the issue of whether or not we ought to believe them. As Glover (2006, 14) argues, first-person accounts and the preferences they reveal need to be interpreted with alertness to possible biases. Dreger, for one, is inclined to take conjoined twins "at their word," but the discussion about normal human functioning suggested that there should be more to our evaluation than sole reliance on first-person accounts. First-person accounts, then, can be interpreted in the light of what we consider to be normal or species-typical functioning.

Moreover, as Glover suggests, "we can draw on a history of reflection on the nature of human flourishing, and on the contribution to it of different aspects of our lives" (2006, 14). With that in mind, it is worth pointing out that the benefits of less individuation or more twin-type behavior are usually associated with having a choice in the matter. Whether or not we "truly are or wish to be independent of others," the idea that it is ultimately our choice is considered to be both typical and desirable. Indeed, cultivating and acting upon our own choices, *on our own* if we so desire, could be said to be central components of a flourishing human life. For conjoined twins, these capacities are restricted. Hence, it is hard to see how conjoined twins are not disabled, at least in these respects.

The importance that we tend to attach to the capacity for free choice and action is illustrative of the need to temper first-person accounts both with consideration about what is normal or species-typical and evaluation with regard to what capacities are important to our flourishing as human beings. All of these things will contribute to our assessment of the impact that specific functional limitations have on a human life. What is also evident from some first-person accounts of being conjoined is that human flourishing is far from an all-or-nothing enterprise. Such accounts persuasively suggest that conjoined twins can lead flourishing lives. They correspondingly suggest that we should be cautious about accepting some of the assumptions lying behind the drive for separation surgery.

However, of crucial importance to our analysis is the fact that we do not need to show, nor should we, that conjunction is not disabling in order to justify caution about separation. Conjunction clearly is likely to be significantly disabling. Thus, to deny that conjoined twins are disabled in any way is the wrong way to go about arguing, if we want to, that separation surgery is not always the best option. As argued above, we might look instead at first-person accounts, at what we consider to be important aspects of a flourishing human life, and at how our analyses might be complicated both by the social aspect of much disability and by the social influence on what we consider to be normal.

Another option is to argue that conjoined twins are, in a sense, a different breed, requiring separate and different evaluations about what is normal and what it is to flourish in their case. It is to this that we now turn.

## THE MORAL-ONTOLOGICAL STATUS OF CONJOINED TWINS

This section looks at the view that the moral and/or ontological status of conjoined twins is importantly different from that of separate twins. For example, it might be claimed that there is something about conjunction that means the twins are not separate persons, or that they are not distinct beings with the individual rights and interests. The orthodox view is that conjunction does not make a fundamental difference to the moral status of the twins, although there are two radically different variants of this orthodoxy.

On the one hand there are those, like Helen Watt, who think even infant conjoined twins are "human moral subjects":

> If by "person"—or "human person"—we mean a human moral subject then this subject is, I would suggest, the human being: the living human organism. We are bodily beings, not purely spiritual beings or series of thoughts. . . . The human moral subject is . . . the underlying bodily being who is the subject of interests and rights. . . . We need to go back to the concept of an organism—a living, self-organising whole—to count how many human organisms were present in the case of *Re A* [conjoined twins]. It was clear from the physical behaviour attributed to Jodie and Mary that there were two separate systems of self-organisation, despite some overlap in the parts controlled by each system. . . . In contrast, where a baby is born with (for example) an extra leg, this leg is not a part of an alternative self-organising system. Rather, it is simply an abnormal part of the baby from whom it is protruding. (2001, 237–38)

On the other hand, there are bioethicists like John Harris who argue that (in the case of infants) neither twin is a person:

> There is something about Mary's life expectancy that makes plausible the decision [to separate] in *Re A* and distinguishes Jodie and Mary [infant conjoined twins] from Gilbert and George [adult conjoined twins]. It is that the life expectancy of Mary between the time when the operation would take place and

her inevitable death, would not have been expectancy of what might be called "biographical life," not the life of a person. Indeed, neither Mary nor Jodie had started living biographical lives, neither were persons properly so called at the time of the operation. On this analysis, the life Mary would lose by the performance of the operation which would kill her, would not have been life from which she could benefit significantly, not life that could ethically be distinguished from her life *in utero*. (2001, 233)

This is not the place to attempt to adjudicate between Watt and Harris, and it will suffice to say that neither differentiates conjoined from other twins. In Watt's view, all are "human moral subjects," while Harris believes none are (if we restrict ourselves to infants). Watt and Harris would also, we presume, agree about mentally competent adult twins: that is, both would assign personhood and moral significance to these, conjoined or otherwise.

## Bratton and Chetwynd's Alternative

Our focus in most of the rest of the paper is on an interesting recent critique of and alternative to this orthodoxy, which can be found in Bratton and Chetwynd's paper "One into Two Will Not Go: Conceptualising Conjoined Twins" (2004). Their paper is critical of the decision to separate Jodie and Mary in *Re A*, a decision which provokes in them a "deep sense of unease" and which they describe as "a startling example of the strong emphasis in the Western ethical and legal tradition on physical separateness as a constitutive feature of individual identity" (279).

The mistake, according to Bratton and Chetwynd, is to think of the conjoined twins as "entangled singletons" who were "intended to be physically separate" (281). This view is problematic, they claim, because "it assumes something about the nature of human individuality (that having a body physically separate from that of others is an essential part of it) that cannot be philosophically justified" (283). Furthermore:

> By treating Jodie and Mary as if they were singletons . . . their lordships tended to resolve the predicament in a way that was detrimental to one of the twins. . . . We argue that separation is detrimental to both twins, since they both lose part of themselves in the process. So conceiving of the twins as singletons both conceives of them as less than they are, and, since it regards separation as the primary aim, tends to ignore the loss to both of them in separation. (281)

The following three major claims are made by Bratton and Chetwynd and each merits scrutiny. First, we ought not to conceptualize conjoined twins as "entangled singletons." Second, following Dreger (1998), we should view being conjoined as part of the twins' "individualities." And third, separation is generally detrimental to both twins because, when separated, they "lose part of themselves" (Bratton and Chetwynd 2004, 281).

## The Entangled Singletons View

A close reading of Bratton and Chetwynd suggests that what they term the "entangled singletons view" involves four distinct elements:

  (a) conjoined twins should be seen as two separate conjoined entities, not as a single entity;
  (b) conjoined twins are or were "intended to be physically separate";
  (c) there is a presumption in favour of separation, and separation is the primary aim of medical intervention;
  (d) physical separateness is essential to individuality. (2004, 283–84)

Taking the first of these first, it should be noted at the outset that asking unqualified "how many entities are there?" questions is liable to be pointless since, in order for quantification questions to make sense, we need to know what *type* of entity is being quantified. This applies just as much to everyday collections of objects, like the contents of people's freezers, as it does to conjoined twins, or indeed to any human beings. It is far from clear, then, that the entangled singletons view, or any other view of conjoined twins, can be characterized in these bare terms—one entity or two?—since we need to know what *type* of entity is at issue. We'll return to this shortly when we look at what Bratton and Chetwynd have to say about "individuals."

The second element, that the twins were "intended to be physically separate," strikes us as a rather odd thing to say, not least because it is not clear who or what is supposed to be doing the intending. In their paper, Bratton and Chetwynd suggest that when people (such as the Law Lords) have an adversarial model of the twins' competing interests, this is (often) because they "think persons are somehow intended or meant to be singletons; that is, physically separate, one person to each body and *vice versa*" (282).

Presumably, they are not referring to parental or divine intentions here, so we can only assume that what they must have in mind is something like the proper functioning of the organism (as in "my heart is meant [intended] to pump blood" or "my legs are meant [intended] for walking"). Thus, an infant human is, in this sense, "intended" to be separate if separateness is required for the proper functioning of its body. If interpreted in this way, it seems to us that (b) is plausible because, as we showed in the first part of this chapter, conjunction normally involves functional impairment.

We find it hard to believe that anyone actually subscribes to the second part of (c), that separation is the *primary aim* of medical intervention. For surely even those who are proseparation will see it not as an end in itself but as a means of achieving some other good, or averting an evil. So perhaps there is some "strawmanning" going on here. As regards the presumption in favor of separation, this seems to us to be defensible and to follow from conjunction's involving impairment. However, it must be emphasized that this presumption in favor of separation could easily be overturned by other considerations, most obviously the health and welfare of the twins (including psychological factors) and, in the case of competent adult twins, the absence of valid consent.

Finally, we turn to the claim that physical separateness is essential to individuality. The fundamental problem with this is that the meaning of "individuality" is obscure. Is an "individual" a person (or protoperson), or an organism, or something else? "Individual" is an inopportune term here, first, because one of its ordinary language meanings is "separate," and so it is not unreasonable to think that separateness is essential to individuality, and second, because (as with the quantification question) the unqualified "is *X* an individual?" is a hopelessly vague question. Indeed, the way Bratton and Chetwynd use the term seems almost to involve some kind of category mistake, as if being an individual were itself being a *particular kind of* thing (or being). In fact, being an "individual" is being one (separate?) thing, the type of which needs to be specified. John, for example, might at the same time be an individual man and father, while also being a collection of (individual) cells and merely a part of his (individual) football team. Thus, issues around "how many individuals?" ultimately collapse into a version of the futile "how many entities?" question.

From this, we can draw some intermediate conclusions. We are looking for a possible alternative view of the moral and/or ontological status of conjoined twins that might impact (at least indirectly) on the permissibility of separation. We have already seen, though, that it is not possible (as Bratton and Chetwynd have tried to do) to characterize this alternative view in terms of unqualified claims about how many entities or how many individuals there are, since claims of this kind are hopelessly vague and perhaps even meaningless. For we need to know what *types of* entity are in question before we make sense of the "how many?" question. So (a) and (d) above, which were supposed to form part of the characterization of the entangled singletons view are incoherent or meaningless. The other elements, (b) and (c), do make sense, but we have argued above that (with some caveats) they are plausible and should be accepted. Therefore, Bratton and Chetwynd's critique of the entangled singletons view seems to be seriously flawed on both these counts.

## Conjunction, Individuality, and Identity

These points about the meaning of "individuality" apply similarly to Bratton and Chetwynd's second and third claims: that we should view being conjoined as part of the twins' "individuality," and that (therefore) both twins would "lose part of themselves" if separated. Let us, however, leave these concerns to one side now and turn to the related idea that separated twins have lost part of themselves, even in cases where separation surgery is otherwise successful. This is an interesting claim for our purposes because, if it were true, it would provide a special (although presumably defeasible) reason for not separating, even where the clinical indications told in favor of separation.

The first thing to say about such phrases as "losing part of themselves" is that they can be read more or less literally, and more often than not they are metaphorical or poetic expressions of an underlying truth which, though important, is much less metaphysically significant than the language might suggest. For example, people who are experiencing grief sometimes say that, in losing a loved one, they have lost part of themselves. But although such talk may powerfully express a profound underlying truth about the meaning and shape of that person's life, the griever has not, we would suggest, *literally* lost a part of herself. Rather, she survives (completely) but has lost an important *aspect* or *part* of her life. So one, quite plausible, approach to Bratton and Chetwynd's claim is to concede that it is true but only in this metaphorical or poetic sense. It powerfully expresses the twins' sense of loss, but they have not literally lost part of themselves.

If this were the correct interpretation, then clearly the claim would be less interesting than it at first appeared, since the psychological harm that it describes could be captured in more mundane terms—and, of course, psychological damage of this kind should be factored into any decision about whether to separate. Taking account of such psychological factors, though, would not require any deviation from the standard principles of clinical ethics and practice—most obviously, concern for the patients' welfare. So if we interpret Bratton and Chetwynd's claim in this metaphorical way, while it may be true (in this special sense), it probably won't have the sort of interesting implications that we seek.

A more literal and stronger interpretation is that being conjoined is *part of the individual essence* of each twin. This "individual essence" claim could be understood as about either identity across possible worlds or identity over time, or both. The "identity across possible worlds" claim is that there are no possible worlds in which A is born in a nonconjoined state, while the "identity over time" claim is that B and C (conjoined twins at time $t_1$) cannot logically survive separation. So if separation surgery took place and two separate children left the operating table at time $t_2$, these children (B\* and C\*) would not be B and C, but rather *replacements for* B and C (who, on this view, would be dead). The relationship between B\* and B would (in the standard case) be very close insofar as B\* was both psychologically and spatiotemporally continuous with B (and C\* with C), but nonetheless (in this view) B\* would not be the same person as B, since conjunction was part of B's individual essence and so logically B cannot survive without it.

This individual essence claim is highly implausible in either interpretation. Taking the first interpretation first, imagine two possible scenarios. In one, an embryo splits at an early stage of development and a pair of nonconjoined twins is born. In the second, the same embryo only partially splits and a pair of conjoined twins is born. According to the individual essence view, different people will result in these two scenarios, even if the same embryo is involved at the outset and there are no other differences between two pairs of twins except for the fact that only one pair separated fully. There seems to us to be no rationale for making this nonidentity claim, and it is not consistent with a number of commonsense things that the twins could think. For instance, cannot the separate twins truly say, "If the embryo hadn't fully separated, we would have been conjoined twins"? And conversely, cannot the conjoined twins truly say, "If the embryo had fully separated, we would have been separate twins"? According to the nonidentity viewpoint, both of these thoughts are false; the correct counterfactual is: if the embryo had (hadn't) fully separated, then we *would not have existed*. Although commonsense intuitions about identity can certainly be wrong sometimes, we should only depart from them if there is a good reason to do so and/or if there is an explanation as to why they are likely to be mistaken. In this case, we can see no such reasons and therefore suggest that the same twins would be born in each of these two possible worlds, conjoined in one case and not in the other.

The second version of the nonidentity claim ("identity over time") is equally implausible. Here, the main idea is that separation is like death because being conjoined is part of the individual essence of each twin. Personal identity over time is a complicated business, and we cannot hope to explain or defend a full account here. Nonetheless, we would contend that where B is both psychologically and spatiotemporally continuous with B*, and where there is no "branching" of either a physical or psychological kind, then B *is* B*. In general terms, this is a highly plausible principle of personal identity over time.[4] Furthermore, it is bolstered in this case by looking at the ethics of separating conjoined twins. As we have seen, on the nonidentity concept, if successful separation surgery took place and two separate children left the operating table, these children (B* and C*) would not be B and C, but rather replacements for B and C. B and C would have been sacrificed in order to bring B* and C* into existence. But if that is the case, then there is no moral difference between separation surgery of the kind just described and a quite different scenario in which B and C are killed and their body parts used to create two new unrelated children, D and E. These two situations are essentially the same, according to the nonidentity view, because in both cases B and C are sacrificed in order to create other children. But since, it seems to us, these two scenarios are morally different (i.e., we hold that, *other things being equal*, separation surgery is less objectionable than killing the twins and harvesting their body parts), we reject the nonidentity view. One response to this argument is simply to "bite the bullet" and claim that separation surgery really is as bad as murdering the conjoined twins and harvesting their organs and that this just goes to show how bad separation surgery is. But we suspect that this is not a line that many writers on conjoined twins would be willing to take.

Finally, we should mention briefly another ethical implication of the nonidentity view. This relates to "sacrifice" cases like the ones discussed by Shel-

don and Wilkinson (1997): ones where B can be saved only if B and C are separated, C will inevitably be killed by the separation, and if no action is taken
C will die in a couple of weeks anyway. In such cases, the nonidentity view
suggests that separating in an attempt to save B will always be wrong, since
B cannot logically be saved by separation, and it will inevitably kill both.
Thus, anyone who believes that sacrifice separations are sometimes permissible has a further reason for rejecting the nonidentity view.

## CONCLUSION

In this chapter we have evaluated two claims. The first says that being conjoined is a "mere difference" rather than a disorder, disability, or impairment.
The second says that conjoined twins have a moral and/or ontological status
that is significantly different from that of other children. We have argued that
both these claims are false, or at least that there are reasons to doubt them.

In rejecting the first claim, we argued that conjunction inevitably involves
some degree of functional impairment and that, in most cases, this will make
human flourishing less likely and hence constitute a disability. It does not
follow from this that separation is always, or even usually, justified. Our
point rather is that to deny that conjoined twins are disabled is the wrong
way to go about arguing for a cautious approach to separation surgery. A
better way would be simply to point out the practical disadvantages of separation, including the psychological ones discussed by Dreger and others.

Our examination of the second claim focused on one particularly clearly articulated version of it, that propounded by Bratton and Chetwynd. Their approach, and more generally views like theirs, seems to contain two fundamental flaws. First, it is not (as they imply) possible to characterize the issue in
terms of unqualified claims about how many "individuals" there are, since
statements of this kind are hopelessly vague and possibly even meaningless.
Second, the idea that being conjoined is part of the identity, or individual
essence, of each twin is highly implausible (for the reasons outlined above). An
alternative way of understanding what Bratton and Chetwynd say about identity is as a psychological claim about the twins' "sense of self." But if read in
this way, we could simply factor identity issues into a *psychological* assessment
of the pros and cons of separation, and there would be no need to posit a fundamental ontological difference between conjoined twins and other children.

## NOTES

1. "Doing something about it" need not imply medical intervention. Removing social disadvantages and/or implementing social provision can render functional limitations relatively, if
not completely, unproblematic.

2. Leaving aside, for now, the question of how "one" can legitimately be described.

3. We are leaving aside the inability to do much *with* the cooperation of a third party since that would seem to depend on particular social structures, conventions, attitudes, and arrangements, which need not directly result from impairment.

4. See Parfit 1984, part 3, for a seminal discussion of these issues.

## REFERENCES

Bratton, M. Q., and S. B. Chetwynd. 2004. One into two will not go: Conceptualising conjoined twins. *Journal of Medical Ethics* 30: 279–85.

Buchanan, A., D. Brock, N. Daniels, and D. Wikler. 2000. *From chance to choice: Genetics and justice.* Cambridge: Cambridge University Press.

Dreger, A. D. 1998. The limits of individuality: Ritual and sacrifice in the lives and medical treatment of conjoined twins. *Studies in the History and Philosophy of Biology and Biomedical Science* 29: 1–29.

———. 2004. *One of us: Conjoined twins and the future of normal.* Cambridge, MA: Harvard University Press.

Glover, J. C. B. (forthcoming). *Choosing children: The ethical dilemmas of genetic intervention.* Oxford: Oxford University Press.

Harris, J. 2001. Human beings persons and conjoined twins. *Medical Law Review* 9 (3): 221–36.

Hull, R. 1998. Defining disability—a philosophical approach. *Res Publica* 4 (2): 199–210.

Parfit, D. 1984. *Reasons and persons.* Oxford: Clarendon Press.

Sheldon, S., and S. Wilkinson. 1997. Separating conjoined twins: The legality and ethics of sacrifice. *Medical Law Review* 5: 149–71.

Watt, H. 2001. Conjoined twins: Separation as mutilation. *Medical Law Review* 9 (3): 237–45.

Wilkinson, S. 2003. Separating conjoined twins: The case of Laden and Laleh Bijani. Cardiff Centre for Ethics, Law and Society, "Issue of the Month," August. http://www.ccels.cardiff.ac.uk/issue/wilkinson.html.

# 7

## ✢

# Conjunction and Separation: Viable Relationships, Equitable Partings

### *David Wasserman*

People speak of couples whose lives are deeply intertwined and interdependent as "joined at the hip." This is usually said affectionately, or at least neutrally, in part because the couples are not literally conjoined. Popular views of those who are literally conjoined are not so favorable. Indeed, critics of the surgical separation of conjoined twins argue that the view of such lives as constricted and undignified often underlies the willingness to risk death and impairment to free conjoined twins from their perceived mutual bondage (Dreger 2004, ch. 2).

The difficulty we congenital "singletons" (a term I use to include unconjoined twins) have in assessing life conjoined may arise in part from our images of temporary conjunction. We are amused by the blundering efforts of discretely embodied individuals in three-legged races and engaged by the drama of escaped convicts shackled to each other, as depicted in such movies as *The Defiant Ones*. So many formerly independent activities, from walking to sleeping, become joint ventures, requiring close coordination. We think that successfully handling such mutual dependence requires a cooperativeness, grace, and empathy for which escaped convicts are not noted. We tend to view the lives of conjoined twins as akin to such passing entanglements, but worse for being permanent. Even in the short term, their lives may seem worse, since conjoined twins have even less choice in their partners than do escaped convicts, and their mutual adaptation may seem only to mitigate an otherwise intolerable confinement. And it must be worse still for twins joined, not at the hip, but at the chest or head, always face to face or never able to achieve direct visual contact.

Disability advocates tend to dismiss such reactions as based on ignorance and hysteria, as reflecting the fear and stigma aroused by anatomical abnormalities, of which conjunction is surely among the most conspicuous. Yet it would be doctrinaire, or naive, to assume that physical conjunction of different types imposes *no* burdens at all on those conjoined; to assume that any burdens not attributable to stigmatization would either be preempted by hard wiring that made conjunction feel utterly natural to those conjoined, or be minimized by a process of adaptation so swift and thorough as to escape notice by those undergoing it. We do know that of those conjoined twins who have lived long enough to express a preference, almost all have said that they wanted to stay conjoined, even when the option of separation was available (Dreger 2004, 43, 46). But we may be a little skeptical of these expressed preferences, not because they reflect denial or false consciousness, but because conjoined twins may find it almost as difficult to imagine living separately as the rest of us find it to imagine living conjoined. Perhaps conjoined twins find the prospect of separation as daunting and oppressive as most of us find the prospect of conjunction. This symmetry is not complete, of course; conjoined twins have grown up surrounded by real and fictional displays of normal, happy singleton lives; the reverse is obviously not true.

Yet the reluctance of conjoined twins to be separated is all the more impressive in light of the hardships they clearly face in being conjoined—not the hardships of finding a modus vivendi for themselves, but the lack of environmental accommodation for human beings configured as they are, and more important, the prejudice and morbid curiosity they constantly face. Their psychological attachment to their physical embodiment must be strong indeed if it holds up against the prospect of escaping that exclusion and that gaze.

In this chapter, I will explore two sets of issues that bear on the justification for separating conjoined twins: the impact of their physical attachment on their well-being, and their rights against each other. These issues may acquire greater relevance as advances in obstetrics and neonatology result in the survival of increasing numbers of conjoined twins, and as advances in surgery make separation a viable option for an increasing number of those twins. In the final section, I will concede that the latter development is likely to limit the practical significance of this inquiry, because the routine separation of conjoined twins at the earliest possible moment may well obviate many of the issues I will raise about the prospects for living well conjoined and the rights arising from different forms of conjoint embodiment.

## WELL-BEING, SHARED EMBODIMENT, AND SEPARATION

The risks of separating conjoined twins have become familiar to newspaper readers, treated with increasingly frequency to detailed accounts of the preparations, procedures, and aftermath (e.g., Lite 2004). Much less is written about the kind of life the twins might lead were they not separated. Often, this is because their conjoined lives are expected to be brief—a few months or years. But the dire forecasts of surgeons eager to operate must be taken with a grain of salt. And in quite a few cases, the alternative to separation, with all its attendant risks, is seen as not death but bondage, the surgery not as life-saving but merely as liberating. If forecasts of early death are suspect, claims about bondage are even more so. Those deciding on the non-emergency separation of conjoined neonates, whether the twins themselves or their surrogates, need a fuller understanding of the kind of lives they are likely to lead if they stay attached.

In decisions on separation, how much weight should be given to the apparent satisfaction of most conjoined twins with their embodiment? There is no reason to receive the positive self-reports of many conjoined twins with any greater skepticism than those of more typically embodied individuals. But this does not mean that we should take their testimony as conclusive evidence of how well they are doing. Because I think that "well-being" is best understood in terms of what philosophers call an "objective list" of valuable activities, capacities, and experiences (e.g., Griffin 1986; Nussbaum 1992), I do not think that conjoined twins—or anyone else, for that matter—will always be right in assessing how well they are doing.

To say that conjoined twins successfully adapt to their embodiment is to describe a psychological process, not to state a normative conclusion. The question remains of whether such adaptation should be regarded as making the best of a bad situation, or as coming to appreciate a good one. In answering this question, however, we should accord great weight to the twins' self-assessments. Because we lack anything close to a complete objective list, or theory, and because, in its absence, we are in constant danger of bias, insularity, and parochialism, we should be reluctant to dismiss or second-guess the self-appraisal of people with lives that differ greatly from our own, culturally or anatomically. Any plausible objective account of well-being must be highly pluralistic, recognizing that people can flourish in a wide variety of ways.

Yet the lives of conjoined twins may appear to test the limits of our pluralism. Their interdependence is, in obvious respects, much greater than that between almost any pair of discretely embodied people.[1] The question is whether this greater interdependence prevents conjoined twins from flourishing as fully as the rest of us can.

A look at the actual lives of some conjoined twins suggests a negative answer—that their differences in physical embodiment, however striking, are compatible with the kind of relationships and activities we value in our own lives. As Alice Dreger observes:

> [A] close reading of the many biographies of conjoined people clearly shows that their lives are not necessarily horrible, unbearable, or even that unusual. Some pairs have lived reasonably long lives. . . . Quite a number have had

lovers, and a few . . . have had children and families. Many have traveled widely, been well educated, enjoyed occupations. Some have had positively boring lives worthy of the most "normal" among us. (2004, 31)

Because lovers, children, families, education, and travel are not merely evidence of flourishing, but partially constitutive of it, Dreger's canvass goes some way toward answering the question of how well conjoined lives can go. Yet it is not a complete answer, for two reasons. First, it does not tell us how common, or how difficult, such success is. Perhaps leading lives of ordinary fulfillment requires extraordinary tenacity, resourcefulness, or luck on the part of conjoined twins. Second, even those lives that appear outwardly successful may have been lived in detail in ways that we would find oppressive or undignified. Our aversions may, of course, reflect nothing more than overly delicate sensibilities, and our interest in the private lives of conjoined twins may be no less voyeuristic than that of the Victorian audiences who paid to have them revealed. Yet the possibility that we will be shown up as prigs or voyeurs should not keep us from examining conjoined lives as closely and critically as we are often urged to examine our own. If we should not be guided by our repugnance, we should not be scared off by it either.

In answering the question of how well conjoined lives can go, then, we need to know something about the details of their lives. But the inquiry is not strictly a factual one; it has a moral, or at least a normative, dimension. Is privacy, for example, a flexible enough notion to encompass the conventions established by conjoined twins for such "intimate" activities as sex and defecation? Can those conventions substitute for the varying degrees of physical isolation that most of us singletons insist on? Or does privacy truly require some degree of physical separation not possible for all or most conjoined twins? And if it does, is it possible to lead a dignified life that lacks privacy, or a life that is dignified overall despite the occasional or frequent indignities that result from the lack of privacy?

The same kinds of questions arise for autonomy as for privacy. Can an individual have a range of life plans large enough to have a meaningful choice among them even if he is limited to plans whose impositions his conjoined twin would accept? May his twin's interests, plans, or activities so encroach on his own that neither can live meaningful and autonomous lives? Does the vulnerability of the life plans of one conjoined twin to the plans, values, preferences, and whims of the other differ only in degree, not kind, from the vulnerability of a singleton's plans?

As Dreger points out (2004, 32–33), these questions cannot be addressed in a social vacuum. The prospects of conjoined twins for privacy and autonomy may depend as much on their social environment as their physical embodiment. It may be, as Dreger suggests, that our own society fetishizes individuality, placing an even heavier burden on conjoined twins than on the rest of us. Moreover, stigma and discrimination may be more formidable barriers to well-being than any physical constraints. But the relevance of the social environment to the appraisal of conjoined lives is complex. If it is taken as a given, which it is for most people most of the time, its oppressive character provides reasons for separation. But if it is seen as mutable, and odious, it provides stronger reasons for social action than for surgery. It will often be hard to decide whether the appropriate response to the barriers imposed by discrimination is acquiescence or defiance.

These questions are similar to the ones that are raised by decisions about interventions for the individual anatomical abnormalities now susceptible to partial or complete medical normalization, from cleft palate to deafness. How well can one live with these conditions, given the physical environment and social attitudes and practices of the society in which one lives? Can parents make the decision to medically normalize their children, at a stage when the medical prospects for normalization are far better, even if there is a good chance that the child, if not normalized, would insist that he would not have wanted to be? To the extent that the burdens associated with the abnormality arise from discrimination and lack of accommodation by society, is medical normalization an inappropriate response, complicit in those social wrongs? Or is it the prerogative of the victims of those wrongs, or their guardians, to seek to avoid or mitigate them? In making these decisions vicariously, it is important to take account of stigma without perpetuating it, without assuming that physical abnormalities are as limiting as they are conspicuous.

## RESOLVING CONFLICTS BETWEEN THE INTERESTS OR DEMANDS OF CONJOINED TWINS

However similar the questions facing conjoined twins and atypical singletons, their resolution will often be more complex for the former. When these questions arise for very young singletons, they can be addressed under the familiar rubric of "the best interests of the child"—the prevailing standard for adjudicating legal disputes about children too young to make their own choices. That standard can be applied to conjoined twins when each faces the same or very similar risks and benefits from separation. For example, the issue of whether separation serves the best interests of conjoined twins by avoiding or mitigating disability discrimination resembles the issue of whether racial matching serves the best interests of minority adoptees by avoiding or mitigating racial discrimination. In considering the best interests of individual children, family law often confronts hard tradeoffs, for example, between preserving parental and sibling relationships and securing a safer, richer, and more stable rearing environment. But the courts generally make those trade-offs separately for each child. In deciding whether it is in a child's best interests to be reunited with her siblings, the court considers only the interest of the child, not of her siblings, in reunification. It is only in cases where the best interests of different siblings, all before the court, are found to conflict, that the courts must explicitly balance those interests.

The best interests of conjoined twins are more likely to conflict, or to be seen as conflicting. Separation or other surgery may benefit one more than the other, or—though this has yet to be seen—it may be sought by one twin but not the other. The differential impact of surgery on conjoined neonates raises vexing problems for the adults who must decide about separation. In some cases, the moral asymmetry of benefit and harm may be decisive: it may appear that no amount of expected benefit to one twin would justify the imposition of significant harm on the other. But claims of rights or ownership will often arise, and those claims may be thought to supersede any balancing of interests. The harm of separation may have less moral weight if the more vulnerable twin has a weaker claim to the resources she would lose. At an extreme, separation can be justified as protecting the twin with a superior claim to the vital organs from their life-threatening usurpation by the other.

As I have argued elsewhere, however, it is not clear how the anatomies of conjoined twins can establish rights to organs under the skin of both (Wasserman 2001). In some cases, organs are situated on one side, or in one body cavity; they are, or appear to be, organs that would have belonged solely to one twin or the other had they not been conjoined. But, at least for organs not under the voluntary control of either twin, the relevance of this counterfactual is not clear. Neither twin ever enjoyed exclusive use of the organs, which have been shared their entire lives. A rule that gave a conjoined twin superior rights to the organs "on its side" or "in its body cavity" might yield determinate results for most organs in most types of conjunction, and its adoption might lead to more cases where at least one twin survived to adulthood. But it would lack a firm moral foundation. Indeed, a reliance on the probable location of organs in separate twins to determine their ownership by conjoined twins involves a figurative normalization, a judicial apportionment of body parts in conformity to a singleton model.

It is not certain if claims of right will be raised more often by older twins than by the surrogates for younger ones. But the former may have greater force, since the strength of claims made by surrogates will be diminished by any uncertainty that they would have been raised by the children themselves. Yet the resolution of the conflicting rights-claims made by older twins may be affected by their prior relationship. They may have reached a more or less explicit modus vivendi, involving complex arrangements for sharing organs and coordinating behavior—arrangements that may be seen as modifying, compromising, or waiving rights they might otherwise been able to assert. Perhaps, to take a simple case, a twin now demanding separation had opposed it at various times when the other twin's prospects for surviving or thriving after the surgery were far better. Or perhaps by merely acquiescing for years in his sibling's use of the organs on his side, the now-complaining twin could be regarded as having lost his exclusive right to those organs, by an extension of the legal doctrine of "adverse possession," which gives legal title to those who openly appropriate others' property for a sufficiently long period of time. But this is uncharted territory, where the law will have to make its way with questionable analogies.

## Balancing the Conflicting Interests and Claims of Conjoined Twins

Because the twins' anatomy and prior arrangements may not establish their rights to disputed body parts, there may be no way to resolve many conflicts about separation on the basis of rights. It may be necessary to balance the twins' interests or claims, and in balancing, it may be hard to resist taking account of their expected quality of life. Thus, in an earlier article (Wasserman 2001, 11), I considered how we should respond to the demands of a 22-year-old, cognitively normal, conjoined twin to be separated from her barely sentient sister, where (1) both would otherwise die within a year; (2) separation would prolong the life of the former twin by at least ten years, but cause the immediate death of the latter; and (3) the vital organs shared by the twins are in the body-cavity of the cognitively normal twin. If there is any doubt that the twins' expected quality of life influences our judgment in cases like this, consider how we would respond to a request for separation from the guardian of a barely sentient 22-year-old twin in a case where *she* had the shared vital organs on her side. I suspect we would be far more inclined to oppose separation in such a case, to see it as unfair to the cognitively normal twin who would lose access to the disputed organs. Indeed, our recognition of rights may be shaped more by the cognitive status of the twins than by their anatomy. We may be more likely to see separation as the killing of a human being when that human being can herself protest the proposed separation in just those terms.

Perhaps we could resist the temptation to base life-and-death decisions on judgments of quality of life, or on doubtful claims of right covertly informed by those judgments, by considering how we would resolve similar conflicts between twins of roughly equal mental and physical capacity or potential. Yet this recourse forces us to confront other difficult issues: should we "privilege" inaction over action, letting nature take its course in cases where the conflicting claims of conjoined twins are of equal strength? Does deference to the biological status quo respect the outcome of a "natural lottery," or does it deny one twin her right to an equal chance for the satisfaction of her equal claim? Should we treat differences in length, but not quality, of life as tie-breakers? If so, how much of a difference in expected length should be required to break a tie? Should we give lexical priority, or only greater weight, to saving or prolonging life over avoiding or correcting impairments? For those who study the ethics of health care allocation, most of these are familiar conundrums. But conflicts among conjoined twins will raise them in particularly stark form, without the comforting belief that we can avoid the dilemmas altogether by preventing the scarcity that gives rise to them.

The moral issues raised by contested separations are not limited to the assessment of the twins' conflicting claims. Their separation involves extraordinarily labor-intensive surgery, utilizing some of the most expensive labor in the health care profession. This is likely to remain the case, for two reasons. First, innovation is far more likely to increase the odds of success than to reduce the cost of the attempt. Second, the idiosyncratic character of most conjunctions, even conjunctions of the same general type, is likely to require very costly improvisation. If separation is sought by both twins, or their surrogates, such costs are likely to be ignored, in light of our familiar reluctance to explicitly ration health care. But in cases where one twin, or her surrogate, opposes separation, those costs are likely to be invoked and given considerable weight.

### Intervention without Separation: Contested Surgery without Conflicting Claims

Disputes peculiar to conjoined twins may not be limited to the issue of separation. With respect to each other, conjoined twins will have a very narrow zone of what Anglo-American law and commonsense morality treat as "self-regarding" behavior, presumed to be the individual's "own business." Laws prohibiting suicide and the use of certain drugs are exceptions, understood as such, and hotly contested morally and legally. But as Kenneth Himma notes (1999), a suicide attempt by one conjoined twin, whose success was sure to cause the other's death as well, would not be seen as self-regarding. The impact of the act on the other twin would be direct in a way that its impact on a spouse or child would not be. (Indeed, in the most common setting in which the actions of one singleton have such a direct impact on another—pregnancy—some jurisdictions have sought to restrict behavior otherwise treated as self-regarding, such as the ingestion of alcohol.)

Could Eng—one of the original, eponymous "Siamese twins"—have gotten an injunction against heavy drinking by his brother Chang, which he reportedly saw as jeopardizing his own health? What if Chang countered that he drank mainly to calm his nerves before or after the public appearances on which Eng insisted? Should conjoined twins who share sexual organs be able to veto each other's sexual partners? Would an individual who had intercourse at the request of one and over the objection of the other commit as serious a crime as one who had intercourse with a protesting singleton? Would the "consenting" twin be guilty of soliciting a sexual assault on the other? What if the two twins differed sharply in their willingness to incur the risks of foreign travel, or rush hour commuting? Would risk aversion prevail even at low or moderate levels of risk?

In resolving some of these disputes, there may be surgical options other than separation: perhaps a shared circulatory or respiratory system can be divided, or an additional organ can be implanted, to give each twin her own. Such surgery, however, may have various costs and risks that are unequally borne by the twins, and there may be different ways of performing the surgery that are unequally beneficial or risky to the two. Further, unlike joint property, which is fully owned by both parties, some parts of the conjoined bodies will appear to belong exclusively to one twin or the other, notably their heads and necks. And, as noted earlier, the twins may appear to have unequal claims to other body parts, such as organs that are fully or largely on one "side" or the other.

Not all difficult cases will involve conflicting interests or choices. There may be cases where the twins have grown so sick of each other that both demand separation even though it is very likely to accelerate their deaths. Would the courts see this as a form of surgeon-assisted suicide, if the odds of early death were sufficiently high? Or would the twins' intent to separate be seen as dominating their knowledge of likely death, so as to make the requested procedure merely reckless rather than suicidal? Would the same kind of paternalism that would prohibit surgery risky to both twins also prohibit surgery risky to only one? For example, what if one, not wanting to "be a burden" on the other, readily consented to separation or other surgery likely to kill him or to harm him far more than it benefited his sibling? We allow adult singletons to undergo risky procedures for their siblings, such as kidney donation, but there presumably are limits to the degree of risk we would find acceptable. Would those limits be even lower for conjoined twins, because of a strong if unwarranted suspicion of undue influence or compromised autonomy? Or would they be even higher, since courts and other decision makers are likely to see the risks of separation as offset for both twins by the supposed benefits of normalization?

## THE EMERGING REALITY: EARLY SEPARATION AS THE NORM

My discussion of the potential conflicts over surgical interventions for conjoined twins may seem fanciful. Conjoined twins are rare, and most conjoined twins born alive do not survive to adulthood. Dreger reports that "estimates of the incidence of conjoined twinning in humans vary from 1 in 25,000 births to 1 in 200,000," that at least 40 percent of conjoined twins are stillborn, and that, of those born alive, 35 percent die within a day (2004, 31). According to a recent article, one of the rarer forms of conjunction, *craniopagus* (joining at the head), occurs in only one out of two million live births, and 80 percent of those twins do not live past their second birthday (Morris 2004). While the survival rate for other types of conjunction is higher, surgical advances may make early separation the "standard of care," even in cases where it cannot be seen as a life-saving procedure. For conjoined twins, the trend toward surgical normalization will be reinforced by the celebrity and public sympathy received, respectively, by the surgeons and their patients (for recent examples, see Carey 2004; Morris 2004; Niedowski 2004). As separation becomes more routine, we may expect to see many more conjoined twins surviving, but fewer surviving conjoined.

Had Chang and Eng been born in contemporary Thailand, they might well have enjoyed a different, lesser celebrity than they in fact did. Instead of being displayed to the king of Thailand and then taken on tour, they might have been flown to Johns Hopkins Hospital for highly publicized surgery by an entrepreneurial star like Benjamin Carson. Or perhaps, given the fairly easy surgical challenge they posed, they would have been separated by a less celebrated surgeon in a more obscure hospital, perhaps even in Thailand. After their successful operation, they would have rapidly faded from public view, leading fairly ordinary lives, perhaps the subjects of a retrospective on their 21st birthdays. Is it insensitive to lament the loss of the more interesting lives they would have led, and more broadly, the loss of diversity that results from this, like other, forms of surgical normalization? It is hard to find much value, or diversity, in early death from overstrained organs, and we should be suspicious of the fascination we take in conjoined twins who live long enough to lead interesting lives. It is too easy to see them as curiosities, or perhaps as offensively, as metaphors for human interdependence.

Moreover, the accommodation of conjoined twins poses a singular challenge. While proponents of "universal design" speak boldly of building to encompass the range of human diversity, they cannot hope to encompass the atypical anatomies of all or most conjoined twins. Because conjoined twins will always be rare, and because there are so many forms of conjunction, it will be virtually impossible to tailor the built environment to all or most of them. Even in a society that respected and valued conjoined twins, their daily lives would involve a degree of improvisation that most of us would find daunting. Perhaps such a challenge should be seen as bracing rather than oppressive, but it would be a mistake to trivialize it.

Yet the separation of conjoined twins often has significant costs to those twins, even when it is done for ostensibly life-saving purposes. One or both frequently die, much sooner than they would have if they remained conjoined, even by the self-serving estimates of the eager surgeons. And those who survive often spend their childhoods in the hospital, continuing the grueling process of surgical normalization. That process is often incomplete, leaving them with a variety of impairments that may require almost as much adaptation as the condition from which they were "liberated." There is also the less tangible loss of a peculiarly intimate connection with a sibling, a loss that will be all too easy to obscure when weighed against the physical benefits of separation. The claim that separation often saves the lives of children who would otherwise die within months or years is itself subject to an important qualification. What if the same ingenuity and resources now devoted to separating conjoined twins went into efforts to prolong and improve their conjoined lives? As far as I know, this is an utterly neglected frontier. But if it were not—if leading institutions such as Johns Hopkins and Great Ormond Street hospitals competed to develop the most effective techniques for strengthening the vital organs of conjoined twins—the need for separation might be dramatically reduced.

I conclude that even if surgical advances make the separation of conjoined twins increasingly safe, they should not make it routine. I agree with Dreger (2004, 73–75) that in cases where waiting does not risk the life of either twin, the presumption should be to defer surgery until the twins can decide for themselves—though, as I noted, the question remains of how to proceed if they do not agree. That presumption can be overcome by a number of factors: by serious threats to the health of one or both twins, by realistic concerns that the manner in which they are conjoined will severely impair their physical or even social development, and perhaps by the likelihood that separation will become riskier or more difficult as they age. But the choice should always be made after careful deliberation, with a lively awareness of the prospects for living well conjoined. That choice should also be made with the understanding that a decision either way may engender profound regret: that twins who remain conjoined may lament a constricted or even tormented childhood, while twins separated in infancy may come to regard their surgery as a cruel amputation, the loss of an intimacy greater than any they can achieve as singletons. The separation of conjoined twins should not be seen as their liberation, but as a course of action fraught with difficult trade-offs.

## NOTE

1. For this reason, it is unfair, if provocative, for Alice Dreger to describe the relationship of a mother to her nursing infant as if it were one between unequally dependent conjoined twins (2004, 17–19). As Dreger is well aware, the mother usually takes on a nurturing role voluntarily, and always temporarily, and the child's relationship to her will gradually become less dependent, although perhaps never fully symmetrical. Even at its height, the physical dependence of the child on its mother is only intermittent: even the most voracious infant merely assumes partial command of her mother's body for a small portion of the day. But the comparison, however limited, does raise the question of the extent to which physical dependence is compatible with well-being—does it become less compatible with greater disparities in need, longer duration, or less voluntary imposition?

## REFERENCES

Carey, Elaine. 2004. Twins face operation. *Toronto Star*, December 15.
Dreger, Alice. 2004. *One of us: Conjoined twins and the future of the normal.* Cambridge, MA: Harvard University Press.

Griffin, James. 1986. *Well-being: Its meaning, measurement, and moral importance*. Oxford: Claredon Press.

Himma, Kenneth. 1999. Thomson's violinist and conjoined twins. *Cambridge Quarterly of Healthcare Ethics* 8 (4): 428–35.

Lite, Jordan. 2004. For the first time, the inside dramatic story of the 17-hour battle to separate conjoined twins. *Daily News* (New York), August 8.

Morris, Deborah. 2004. Two brains, one major challenge: Surgeons navigate a risky stage-by-stage procedure designed to give brothers, joined at the head, a chance at separate, healthy lives. *Newsday*, July 18.

Niedowski, Erika. 2004. One girl survives separation surgery. *Baltimore Sun*, September 17.

Nussbaum, Martha. 1992. Human functioning and social justice: A defense of Aristotelian essentialism. *Political Theory* 20 (2): 202–46.

Wasserman, David. 2001. Killing Mary to save Jodie: Conjoined twins and individual rights. *Philosophy and Public Policy Quarterly* 21 (1): 9–14.

# IV

# LIMB AND FACE TRANSPLANTATION

Ethical Issues in Limb Transplants
*Donna Dickenson and Guy Widdershoven*

Changing Faces: Ethics, Identity, and Facial Transplantation
*Françoise Baylis*

# 8

✛

# Ethical Issues
# in Limb Transplants

## Donna Dickenson and Guy Widdershoven

In April 1999, the *Lancet* published an Early Report on the six months' re-sults of the first human hand allograft performed in Lyon in September 1998.[1] The same clinical team performed a double human hand allograft in January 2000. In the interim, a U.S. team at Louisville performed a sim-ilar procedure. Yet permission to perform further human hand allografts has again been refused by the St. Mary's Hospital Trust Clinical Ethics Committee, on which one of the authors sits (DD). Following face-to-face evaluation of hand function in the transplant recipient six months after the operation, the committee reiterated its concerns that the level of func-tion attained did not outweigh the risk. Doubts about "the ethics of put-ting a patient through toxic immunosuppressive therapy for a non-vital operation" were also raised in a commentary on the *Lancet* report.[2] The recipient of the first hand transplant has recently announced that he is actually seeking to have it amputated, saying, "I've become mentally de-tached from it."[3] This article explores the ethical arguments both for and against limb transplant, and particularly human hand allograft, with em-phasis on the issues concerning identity which can be seen in the recipi-ent's reaction.

On one view, hand transplants cross technological frontiers but not ethical ones. They raise no ethical questions that have not been answered long since, in favour of transplantation. There can be no objections except from unre-generate opponents of progress in science—according to one of the very few

Reprinted from Dickenson, Donna and Guy Widdershoven, "Ethical Issues in Limb Trans-plants," *Bioethics*. Reprinted with permission from Blackwell Publishing.

articles in medical ethics to have appeared on the issue of limb transplants. The article concludes in favour of cadaveric hand transplantation, provided professional and procedural standards of competence have been met (including field strength of the clinical team, scientific background of the innovation, and open public evaluation).[4]

Nonetheless, it is broadly agreed that doctors are not obliged to do everything which is technologically possible. We can stave off the moment of death over and over again in terminally ill patients, but there is a widespread dread of pointless "high-tech" intervention. Modern medicine tends to generalise the application of technologically innovative procedures beyond their original target group, as epitomised by the widespread overuse of cardiopulmonary resuscitation.[5,6] Specifically in transplant surgery, "in every instance, the extension . . . to organs beyond the original kidney, such as the heart, liver, lungs and pancreas, has raised questions and controversies in the mind of physicians and the general public."[7] Are limb transplants a step too far down a slippery slope?[8]

Surprisingly little attention has been paid to possible ethical problems in limb transplants. Perhaps this is partly a function of what one study has identified as an "ethics gap" between the medical and surgical literatures in their coverage of biomedical ethics.[9] Some concepts from conventional biomedical ethics may help us elucidate these particular surgical dilemmas: the boundaries of research, burdens and benefits, and patient autonomy.[10] But we will also introduce another set of more speculative and philosophically challenging concepts, which go beyond the scope of conventional biomedical ethics, in order to do justice to some of the unexpected questions that arise in limb transplantation. This second set of issues includes bodily integrity, unnaturalness, and personal identity.

## RESEARCH BOUNDARIES, BURDENS AND BENEFITS, AND PATIENT AUTONOMY

Unlike life-saving transplants, the benefits of limb transplants do not self-evidently surpass the burdens. The risks of lifelong immunosuppressive medication, as well as the possible development of melanomas and other cancers, mean that a limb transplant may actually shorten life. It has been said of medicine that "the art's most delicate aspect is not to shorten life further, and not to diminish it."[11] Other innovative transplant procedures, such as multi-organ transplants, may be criticised as having such unacceptably high mortality rates that they are properly characterised as more research than therapy, and possibly nontherapeutic research at that. Both the case of four-year-old Laura Davies and the two American pediatric cases described by Friedman[12] bear out this ethical qualm, with extensive lymphoma at autopsy in the latter cases.

One might want to argue, however, that medical science only advances by performing procedures at the limit of current knowledge. In that case, limb transplants would be more like research than therapy, and one could expect the risk-benefit ratio to be different. However, the Lyon and Louisville recipients clearly understood the procedure to be therapy, not research. Nor was this supposed research properly designed and evidentially sound. Simply because a procedure is new and unproven does not make it "experimental" or "research." In any case, the standard for subjects' informed consent to participation in medical research is actually higher than for their agreement to therapeutic procedures.[13]

If limb transplants are not to be judged by research standards, the cost-benefit equation which they entail must be considered under the rubric of therapeutic interventions. The most obvious benefit of most other organ transplants, saving life, does not apply to limb transplants. The nearest similarity is to restoration of function, for example, through corneal transplants. However, artificial limbs currently provide a better level of function than the limb transplants so far performed, which does not hold for corneal transplants.

But who should decide on the acceptability of the cost-benefit equation? Here we would normally need to consider both resource allocation—e.g. the expense to the UK National Health Service of lifelong immunosuppressive medication—and benefits to the individual patient. In the case of the Lyon patient, who was paying privately for his own treatment, there was no public resource allocation question (except perhaps insofar as the UK surgeon's time was being diverted away from NHS patients). So the issue resolved itself into a matter of patient autonomy, the third question on our list. The obvious patient autonomy argument in the case of an adult patient is that it is up to the patient to weigh the risks and benefits. If he chooses to accept the risks of an actually decreased life span, his autonomy deserves respect. But why?

Many people would phrase their answer in terms of "whose body is it?", a liberal argument founded loosely on John Locke's assertion in *An Essay Concerning Human Understanding* that "Every man hath a property in his own person." But Locke follows that sentence with another which ought to give us pause: "The labour of his body, and the work of his hands, we may say, are properly his." Locke says we own our labour, not our bodies. And we own our labour because it is the product of our moral agency, which is much closer to what Locke means by "person" than is the physical body.[14,15]

In Locke's terminology, we own that with which we have mixed our labour. It is not literally mixing our bodies with natural resources which gives us a claim to property; that would be an incoherent metaphor. As Robert Nozick has famously pointed out in his fantastical example of pouring his tin of tomato juice into the sea and then claiming he owns the oceans of the world,[16] mixing one substance which I own with another which I do not possess does not make the second one mine. Similarly, it is not the physical contact between my body and the hoe or the land which entities me to claim the harvest. If there is anything special about my work, it is not that it is the labour of my body, but that it represents my agency, a part of my self, my person.

Anglo-American common law views tissue taken from the body not as the property of the person from whose body it comes, but as *res nullius,* no one's property. What the law was traditionally concerned with was making sure that the tissue was not taken without consent, not with what happened to it afterwards; after all, it was presumed to be diseased. Of course we need not literally own our bodies to have rights over their inviolability; indeed, this is closer to the conventional position in law. Common law is more concerned with protecting the physical person from assault or other trespass, through the cornerstone of consent, than with establishing property rights in the body. But this is primarily a negative right, to be free of trespass to the person—not a positive right to demand any and all forms of procedure which I may think desirable.[17] So it is simply not good enough to say that I own my body and can request that whatever I like should be done to it.

Is the argument from autonomy more to do with the right to harm oneself if one chooses? We accept that argument in other procedures involving self-harm, such as donation of a kidney by a living donor. But where do we draw the line about self-harm? Donation of a kidney by a living donor entails a clear benefit to the recipient. What about the recent furore about amputation of healthy limbs to "cure" victims of rare body dysmorphic disorders?[18] These patients have an obsessive belief that their body is incomplete with four limbs, but will be complete after amputation. Here there is no benefit to another person, but the surgeon who performed these procedures felt that he was justified by the threats of suicide or self-harm which these patients had made. (In one case, the patient had already asked a friend to shoot off one of her limbs.) Should we say that amputating healthy limbs is *prima facie* wrong—or at least, not part of the goals of medicine? After all, it carries unpleasant connotations of emotional blackmail, and of colluding with the patient's delusions.

That there should be a class of procedures which are *prima facie* wrong, even if patients request them, seems plausible. It is the underpinning notion behind mental health legislation, after all, that people's motives and desires are not always to be taken at face value. This is not just a matter of the law's distinction between the competent adult's *refusal* of treatment, which may occur on any grounds, or no grounds,[19] and the absence of a right to *request* whatever procedure one wants, although that is part of it. In more philosophical terms, the problem of other minds may mean that the clinician cannot ever fully understand the patient's motives for consenting to, refusing, or requesting a procedure; but that does not mean that the clinician has to conclude that the patient's desires must always be respected.[20]

Let us assume, then, that there is a class of procedures which it would be *prima facie* wrong for the clinician to propose (whether or not the patient agreed) and wrong for the patient to request. If there is a class of procedures which are *prima facie* wrong to perform, what is in that class? Amputation of healthy limbs, in the absence of other justification than that so far encountered, is such a procedure, we suggest. The burden of proof is on the clinician who proposes it, or the patient who requests it, to show why it is not wrong, if further argumentation can be produced. But what about gender reassignment? Somehow that now seems more acceptable, but why? How do we know that the content of the class is not simply down to newness, strangeness, or the "yuck" factor?

For our purposes, we only need to establish that the patient autonomy argument does not trump all. It may be wrong to take advantage of another's willingness to harm himself: motives are complex creatures.[21] Following extensive media coverage of a total artificial heart transplantation in 1982, some volunteers were even willing to "donate" their hearts in the interests of advancing science, though they had no cardiac pathology.[22] In the hand transplant case, the risk is not necessarily certain death, and the benefit of the procedure is to the person undertaking the risk; but there may still be a distinction between respecting the patient's "right" to harm himself and being the agent of possible harm. In interviewing the Lyon recipient, the St. Mary's ethics committee was struck by evidence of possible thought disorder: he denied that his own arm, which had been reattached but failed to "take," was really his, whilst he strongly believed that he would eventually find his "own" arm again when an allograft was performed. With the hand showing signs of rejection two years later because of his failure to take immunosuppressive medication consistently, he now says, "As it began to be rejected, I realized that it wasn't my hand after all."[23] Perhaps he failed to take his immunosuppressive medication precisely because he was under the delusion that the transplanted arm was his own long-lost limb.

How much room is there for critical examination of the patient's motives? The answer to this question depends on how one conceives of autonomy and the interaction between doctor and patient. Emanuel and Emanuel[24] define four models of the doctor-patient relationship:

1. The paternalistic model, in which the doctor knows best;
2. The informative model, in which the doctor merely conveys information and the patient decides;
3. The interpretative model, in which the doctor acts as a counselor or adviser, helping the patient to clarify values;
4. The deliberative model, in which the doctor acts as a friend or teacher, eliciting the patient to critically examine his or her values in a process of communication and deliberation.

In the Lyon case, the surgeons seem to have followed the informative, legalistic model. The patient was asked to sign a detailed consent form and a legal contract, detailing risks in surgery and anaesthesia together with post-surgical risks of possible drug-related complications, malignancies, infections, and long-term psychological complications.[25] The surgical team certainly gave the recipient enough information by the usual professional standards, and indeed more than enough to satisfy the rather minimal requirements of English law.[26] Yet one may doubt the scientific basis of the information given, and therefore the validity of the informed consent. As hand allograft is an "experimental" procedure, there is an insufficient body of evidence on the basis of which patients can be informed. The team in Louisville chose to give the patient a reduced dose of immunosuppressive medication, reasoning that "because a hand transplant is not a life-saving procedure, the drug treatment will be less aggressive than that of other organ transplants."[27] It is not clear whether the U.S. recipient consented to receive a "riskier" treatment regime, and if he did, on what evidential basis.

The interpretative and deliberative models imply that the surgeons should actually focus on the patient's reasons for wanting a hand allograft, given the risks involved. In the Lyon case, this raises some interesting questions. For nearly ten years, following the reamputation of his right forearm after an initial replantation failed, the recipient had refused an aesthetic or functional prosthesis. Was there an element of inability to accept the loss of his hand, and the failure of its replantation? The deliberative model draws our attention to such questions: patient autonomy is not a catch-all answer in this view, but rather the beginning of a questioning process. "The conception of patient autonomy is moral self-development; the patient is empowered not simply to follow unexamined preferences or values, but to consider, through dialogue, alternative health-related values, their worthiness, and their implications for treatment."[28] Of course, there is a considerable risk of slipping over into the paternalistic model here: of overbearing doctors overriding the patient's own values, rather than helping to draw them out. In limb transplants, however, where the motives may be complicated and the benefits might actually be outweighed by the harms, that seems much less of a risk than the converse: failing to examine the patient's decision jointly.

Let us review the issues raised thus far, and evaluate their impact on the ethical status of limb transplants. In this section we have raised three possible ethical objections to human hand allograft in particular:

1. *Is this therapy or research?* The "defence" claimed that limb transplants are research, not therapy, and that they should be allowed because research pushes the boundaries of scientific knowledge forward. The fact that limb transplant is not (yet) a treatment of proven efficacy, however, does not make it research. So this objection still stands.

2. *Do the costs outweigh the benefits?* Even if limb transplants are not *prima facie* wrong to perform, they could be proven wrong with more extensive argumentation, most obviously cost-benefit analysis. In therapeutic treatment, the benefits to the patients should outweigh the possible risks and harms (which would not necessarily be true in research). However, limb transplant is not a life-saving therapy. This is the calculus on the benefit side; on the harm side we have lifelong immunosuppressive medication, which also carries heavy resource implications. In the view of our clinical ethics committee, the degree of function regained did not counterbalance the costs.

3. *Should the patient be the one to decide on the risk-benefit equation?* We might want to argue that it is the patient who should decide what risks are acceptable. If this is so, it is not so because patients straightforwardly own their bodies. The law has traditionally been concerned with protecting patients from unauthorised trespass to the person, but has been unwilling to say that doctors must go along with whatever trespass patients do authorise. There are some procedures which we want to view as outside the goals of medicine, whether the doctor or the patient proposes them. So we come back again to the question of whether limb transplants are among those procedures.

On balance, so far, drawing on all three of the "standard" arguments from bioethics, we have yet to show positive reasons why limb transplants should be performed. Can more unconventional arguments take us beyond this impasse?

## BODILY INTEGRITY AND PERSONAL IDENTITY

Our first set of considerations was fairly standard bioethical fare, although the application to limb transplants is new. The second set is more speculative, but possibly more powerful. So far, we have two "no" results against limb transplants, and one "not proven." The more speculative arguments, in our view, actually favour limb transplants more than the standard ones; but they also require the clinician to take into account some new and unusual factors.

First, bodily integrity: an obvious issue in physiological terms is that invasion of bodily integrity precipitates the immune system's natural reaction, and the consequent need for lifelong immunosuppressive therapy. But the issue is not only biological; it is also symbolic, as is clear from the Lyon team's decision to attempt to restore the normal appearance of the dead donor through a prosthesis—in order, as they put it, to restore the dignity of the donor. That the surgical team felt such a need itself suggests that they felt all was not right. But what exactly is the ethical importance of bodily integrity, and how does it bear on the rightness or wrongness of limb transplants?

The symbolic importance of bodily integrity may explain the emphasis put upon obtaining consent of family members for organ transplants, contrary to the general principle in English law that no one, not even a relative, can give or withhold consent on behalf of an adult patient.[29] In the absence of consent from the patient, bodily integrity is normally sacrosanct. However, the Human Tissue Act 1961 requires doctors to consult relatives about organ donation if there was no previous consent from the deceased person. French law in relation to organ donation is based on the "opt-out" principle; but in the UK, where the "opt-in" system applies, consent must have been obtained from donors before their death. The position is complex in law, but essentially a spouse or relative has the power of veto.[30] In countries with the "opt-out" system, it is also customary to request the relatives' permission, although this too carries no legal weight.[31] Since 1987, U.S. doctors have been required by law to request relatives' permission for "harvesting" organs of deceased patients who had not given a consent before death. Similarly in the Netherlands, a law has recently been enacted which gives patients the option of consenting or refusing donation of their own accord, or of leaving the decision to surviving relatives.

In passing, it is also important to note that the current donor card system in the UK may not cover limb transplants. The card reads:

I request that after my death
A. any part of my body be used for the treatment of others [tick box], or
B. my kidneys [tick box], corneas [tick box], heart [tick box], lungs [tick box], liver [tick box], pancreas [tick box] be used for transplantation.

The donor could be excused for thinking that the list under B covers all parts of the body which can be donated. If so, then ticking A would not imply consent to donating limbs.

We have seen that the law gives an unusual level of power to relatives of organ donors, and that this may be linked to feelings about bodily integrity of the deceased. But there is another possibility, which raises an argument from unnaturalness. Is there a lingering sense among the Western general public that transplantation is somehow unnatural and wrong? This is a view which certainly persists in other cultures such as Japan.[32]

All medical intervention is unnatural in that it constitutes interference with the natural order, although it is perfectly natural in the sense that we are ourselves part of that order.[33] (It may be that the argument from unnaturalness fulfills our need to maintain boundaries against which our choices have value;[34] but this says nothing about where the boundaries should be set.) One argument in favour of xenotransplants has been that all transplants are unnatural, and may affect our sense of bodily integrity, but that our human identity is not wrapped up in any of our organs. "If the essence of humanity is seen as a capacity to transcend their level of organic existence, then a person's sense of identity should not, in theory, be threatened by a transfer of organs across species boundaries," the Nuffield Council Working Party on Xenografts argued.[35]

If this is true of non-human organs, then *a fortiori* it should be true of any human transplant, whether of kidney, limb, or brain tissue. Yet there are two grounds for doubting whether it is true of human transplants. The first is the empirical evidence from transplant recipients, many of whom do report feeling disturbed at the sense of "otherness" of part of a dead person's body in their own.[36] In principle, at least, this could be controlled through psychiatric testing and counseling of recipients. The more challenging question is philosophical: whether some organs, such as the hand, represent personal identity in a way that other organs do not. This leads into a third set of considerations, concerning personal identity.

Opponents of brain tissue transplants often fear that the procedure alters the recipient's identity in a profoundly problematic way—so that the person who gave consent to receiving the tissue is no longer the same person after the transplant.[37,38] Similarly, we need to consider the wider function of the hand in relation to identity, as an instrument of physical intimacy, of contact with others, of consummate skill in artists and musicians, of agency itself—as witness the use of "hand" to represent agency in such phrases as "the hand of Fate," "by his own hand," "the hand of God." The hand plays an unrivaled part in both shaping and standing for the story of both the recipient and the donor, in representing agency, and our language reflects this role.

It might be argued that hand allografts entail the transposition of an organ with personal qualities from one person to another. This goes beyond the issue of the hand's visibility, though that too is an issue. "It may not be easy to live with a transplanted hand, which, unlike other common transplants, remains constantly in full view"[39]—a constant threat to the recipient's sense of his or her own psychological wholeness, arguably outweighing the physical wholeness for which the transplant was sought in the first place. An artificial hand or limb might arguably have the same effect, but on the other hand, there may be a crucial psychological difference. The recipient is not expected to believe that the artificial limb is his or her own, or another person's. There are no personal qualities to be transposed from one to another.

Personal identity, like bodily integrity, has a symbolic character: a person is not only a physical unity, but also a symbolic unity, presented towards others. The French philosopher Ricoeur calls this second notion of identity *ipse*, distinguishing it from the spatiotemporal *idem*.[40] Personal identity as *ipse* is created through interpersonal relations, built upon social practices and shared Stories.[41] This kind of identity is not spiritual: it is embodied. Eminently expressive parts of the body, like the face and hand, represent this identity and the relationships with others which are implied in it. If such body parts are inserted into a completely different context, personal identity is at stake, and so are the interpersonal relationships connected with it.

Likewise, it may be conceivable that the intimacy which the hand can express is transformed as a result of transplantation, necessarily having an emotional impact on those who are intimately related to both donor and recipient. It is indeed unsettling to think that the hand with which one has once been intimate may now stroke another body. Even more than the issue of bodily integrity, the issue of personal identity seems to require extensive communication with close relatives in the case of limb transplantation. But is this enough? Perhaps what we really want to say is that the strangeness of hand transplants has nothing to do with their "experimental" status, or with the "yuck" factor, but with all that the hand represents. The hand occupies a privileged position, as the expression of both agency and intimacy—of our self and our relation to others.

Yet what is so morally special about intimacy? After all, someone like John Harris might argue, having someone to be intimate with is just a form of privilege, like having children. (Harris does not think we should give preference in allocating scarce resources of organs to those who have dependent children.)[42] One of us has argued elsewhere[43] that this is to view children merely as a consumer good, as a possession; the similar point here is that a view like Harris's is impoverished, and an inaccurate representation of how we come to be agents in the first place. It is through social contact, including the contacts of intimacy, that we become moral agents, on accounts which range from Aristotle's to Hegel's, and on into modern narrative, communitarian, feminist, and hermeneutic perspectives. This gives intimacy a claim of precedence on our moral judgment. To the extent that the hand symbolises intimacy, it also gives the hand a special status.

The issues raised in this second section have been less standard and more speculative; or perhaps it is more accurate to say that they have less to do with principlist bioethics and more to do with a narrative or hermeneutic style of ethics, which focuses on the construction and symbolic representation of identity. What conclusions do they suggest?

1. *Symbolic importance of the donor's bodily integrity:* It is difficult to see that limb donation offends against the symbolic importance of bodily integrity any more than does soft tissue donation; the only difference is that it is more visible. However, it is by no means clear that the donor card system includes limbs, and there might be a valid challenge to any presumed consent from relatives. In law, at least, limb transplants might in fact be wrong to perform, without clear and unambiguous consent from the donor.

2. *The argument from unnaturalness:* This, too, appears to fail. All transplants are unnatural; and what is unnatural is neither good nor bad, merely unnatural. So there is no objection to limb transplants on grounds of unnat-

uralness. The effect of this, however, is merely to confirm our initial hypothesis that limb transplants are not *prima facie* wrong to perform, rather than to provide a positive justification for them.

3. *Personal identity and intimacy:* Although these are the most abstract and perhaps speculative grounds for doubting the rightness of hand transplants, they are rooted in a view of human agency which has long historical roots and active current offshoots. The hand, as an expression of both agency and intimacy, occupies a different place in our moral sensibility than internal organs. Again, this is not a reason for absolutely prohibiting hand transplants, if those intimate with both donor and recipient consent, but it is a reason for thinking that the decision is not down to the individual donor or recipient alone.

## CONCLUSION

Is it right to perform limb transplants, and in particular hand allografts? Several of our six criteria merely ratify our initial hypothesis that it is at least not wrong to do so. Two—bodily integrity and intimacy—cast rather more doubt on our hypothesis that limb transplant is not forbidden. Overall, we do not rule out hand allograft *a priori*: transplantation may be consistent with respect for the bodily integrity of both donor and recipient, and the recipient may be able to integrate the new limb into his or her personal identity in a satisfactory way. This will, however, require a great deal of effort from all involved, including family members of both donor and recipient. Our discussion shows that limb transplants are not ethically straightforward: rather, they pose deep ethical dilemmas about autonomy and identity, which certainly cannot be solved by concentrating only on professional standards of competence.

## NOTES

1. J. M. Dubernard, E. Owen, G. Herzberg, M. Lanzetta, X. Martin, H. Kapila *et al*. Human Hand Allograft: Report on the First 6 Months. *The Lancet* 1999; 353: 1315–20.

2. G. Foucher. Commentary: Prospects for Hand Transplantation. *The Lancet* 1999; 353: 1286–87.

3. C. Hallam, quoted in: "Man with New Hand Doesn't Want It," *International Herald Tribune*, 21–22 October 2000, p. 5.

4. M. Siegler. Ethical Issues in Innovative Surgery: Should We Attempt a Cadaveric Hand Transplantation in a Human Subject? *Transplantation Proceedings* 1998; 30: 2779–82, at 2782.

5. M. Hilberman, J. Kutner, D. Parsons, D. J. Murphy. Marginally Effective Medical Care: Ethical Analysis of Issues in Cardiopulmonary Resuscitation (CPR). *Journal of Medical Ethics* 1997; 23: 361–67.

6. P. N. E. Bruce-Jones. Resuscitation Decisions in the Elderly: A Discussion of Current Thinking. *Journal of Medical Ethics* 1997; 22: 286–91.

7. E. Friedman. Editorial: The Desperate Case: CARE (Costs, Applicability, Research, Ethics). *JAMA* 1989; 261: 1483–90.

8. B. Williams. 1985. Which Slopes are Slippery? In: Lockwood M. (ed.) *Moral Dilemmas in Modern Medicine*. Oxford. Oxford University Press: 126–37.

9. F. Paola, S. S. Barten. An "Ethics Gap" in Writing About Bioethics: A Quantitative Comparison of the Medical and the Surgical Literature. *Journal of Medical Ethics* 1995; 21: 84–88.

10. D. Dickenson, N. Hakim. Ethical Issues in Limb Transplants. *Postgraduate Medical Journal* 1999; 75: 513–15.

11. C. Elliott. Doing Harm, Living Organ Donors, Clinical Research, and The Tenth Man. *Journal of Medical Ethics* 1995; 21: 91–96.

12. *Op. cit.*, note 7.

13. J. Montgomery. 1997. *Health Care Law*. Oxford: Oxford University Press: 344.

14. J. Waldron. 1988. *The Right to Private Property*. Oxford: Clarendon Press.

15. D. Dickenson. 1997. Property, Women and Politics: Subjects or Objects? Cambridge: Polity Press.

16. R. Nozick. 1974. *Anarchy, State and Utopia*. New York: Basic Books.

17. *R. v.* Secretary of State for Social Services, W. Midlands AHA & Birmingham AHA (Teaching), *ex parte* Hincks [1980] 1BMLR 93; *R. v.* Cambridge HA, *ex parte* B [1995] 2 All ER 129 (CA); [1995] 1 FLR 1055 (QBD).

18. G. Seenan. Healthy Limbs Cut Off at Patients' Request. *Guardian*. 1 February 2000: p. 9.

19. Re T [1992] 4 All ER 649.

20. Re J [1991] 3 All ER 930.

21. We have excluded discussion of the profit motive in donors, for reasons of space limitation. For further discussion of paid organ donation and "rewarded gifting" (in the context of other organs than limbs), see, *inter alia*: R. R. Bollinger. Ethics of Transplantation. D. J. Rothman, E. Rose, T. Awaya, *et al*. The Bellagio Task Force Report on Transplantation, Bodily Integrity and the International Traffic in Organs. *Transplantation Proceedings* 1997; 29: 2739–45; C. A. E. Nickerson, J. D. Jasper, D. A. Asch. Comfort Level, Financial Incentives and Consent for Organ Donation. *Transplantation Proceedings* 1998; 30: 155–59; A. S. Dear. Guest Editorial: Paid Organ Donation—the Grey Basket Concept. *Journal of Medical Ethics* 1998; 24: 265–368.

22. M. Shaw (ed.). 1984. After Barney Clark: Reflections on the Utah Artificial Heart Program. Austin: University of Texas Press.

23. See note 3.

24. E. J. Emanuel, L. I. Emanuel. Four Models of the Physician-Patient Relationship. *JAMA* 1992; 267: 2221–26.

25. *Op. cit.*, note 1, 1316.

26. Sidaway *v.* Bethlem RHG [1985] 1 All ER 643.

27. Dr. Jon Jones, quoted in *The Guardian*, 26 January 1999.

28. See reference 24, 2222.

29. Re T [1992] 4 All ER 627.

30. For further detail, see: J. Montgomery. 1997. *Health Care Law*. Oxford: Oxford University Press: 427–30.

31. B. W. Haag, F. P. Stuart. 1989. The Organ Donor: Brain Death, Selection Criteria, Supply and Demand. In: M. W. Flye (ed.) *Principles of Organ Transplantation*. Philadelphia: WB Saunders Co.: 185.

32. J. R. McConnell. The Ambiguity About Death in Japan: An Ethical Implication for Organ Procurement. *Journal of Medical Ethics* 1999; 25: 322–24.

33. J. Hughes. Xenografting: Ethical Issues. *Journal of Medical Ethics* 1998; 24: 18–24.

34. R. Norman. Interfering with Nature. *Journal of Applied Philosophy* 1996; 13: 1–11.

35. Nuffield Council on Bioethics. *Animal-to-Human Transplants: The Ethics of Xenotransplantation*. 1996; London. Nuffield Council: 104.

36. J. Craven, G. M. Rodin. 1992. *Psychiatric Aspects of Organ Transplantation*. New York: Oxford University Press: 169–71.

37. G. Northoff. Do Brain Tissue Transplants Alter Personal Identity? Inadequacies of Some "Standard Arguments." *Journal of Medical Ethics* 1996; 22: 174–80.

38. L. Burd, J. M. Gregory, J. Kerbeshian. The Brain-Mind Quiddity: Ethical Issues in the Use of Human Brain Tissue for Therapeutic and Scientific Purposes. *Journal of Medical Ethics* 1998; 24: 118–22.

39. *Op. cit.*, note 2, 1286.

40. P. Ricoeur. 1991. Narrative Identity. In: D. Wood (ed.) On *Paul Ricoeur: Narrative and Interpretation*. London: Routledge: 188–99.

41. G. A. M. Widdershoven. 1993. The Story of Life: Hermeneutic Perspectives on the Relationship Between Narrative and Life History. In: R. Josselson, A. Lieblich (eds.) *The Narrative Study of Lives*. Vol. 1. Newbury Park: Sage: 1–20.

42. J. Harris. 1985. *The Value of Life*. London: Routledge: 105.

43. D. Dickenson. 1991. *Moral Luck in Medical Ethics and Practical Politics*. Aldershot: Gower.

# 9

# Changing Faces:
# Ethics, Identity, and
# Facial Transplantation

*Françoise Baylis*

In September 1998, a team of doctors in Lyon, France, performed the world's first hand transplant (Dubernard et al. 1999; Dubernard et al. 2000). Even as the scientific and lay media celebrated this astonishing technical achievement, however, the attention of some was already focused on the next likely breakthrough—facial transplantation, with hand transplantation cited as proof-of-principle (BBC 1998; Hettiaratchy and Butler 2003). Media interest in human facial transplantation research grew particularly intense in early 2003 when, in Britain, considerable efforts were made by the media to identify the possible recipient of the world's first face transplant (Dougherty 2003).

In response to the increased media attention focused upon facial transplantation, and concerns expressed by the charity Changing Faces, the Royal College of Surgeons of England established a working party to review the science and ethics of facial transplantation. In November 2003, the Royal College issued a report concluding that it would be premature to proceed with human facial transplantation "until there is further research and the prospect of better control of . . . complications" (Royal College of Surgeons 2003, 20). Not long thereafter, in March 2004, the French National Consultative Bioethics Committee decided that it would be unethical to proceed with facial transplantation because of the inherent risks (CCNE 2004). Later that same year, in October 2004, an Institutional Review Board (i.e., research ethics committee) at the Cleveland Clinic in Ohio formally approved a research proposal to remove the face of a cadaver and transplant it onto a person with a severe facial deformity (Cleveland Clinic Foundation 2004; CBS 2004).

Facial transplantation is proposed as a future alternative treatment for persons with serious facial disfigurements resulting from accidents (e.g., severe burns, gunshot wounds), disease (e.g., cancer, severe infections), or congenital birth defects. At present, depending upon the nature of the disfigurement, treatment options include surgical reattachment of the original tissue; autologous transplantation of tissue flaps and skin grafts from other parts of the patient's body (e.g., back, arm, or buttock); and use of prosthetic materials to replace missing tissue. Unfortunately, the outcome of these surgeries is usually disappointing in terms of appearance and function, and frequently there are significant psychosocial sequelae. The hope (expectation) with facial transplantation is that surgeons will be able to improve on cosmetic appearance and mobility.

The proposed transplant will involve at least two surgical teams and three separate surgeries: one surgery to remove the face from the dead donor (i.e., the skin, the underlying fat, and possibly even the entire facial-muscle structure); one surgery to remove the face of the person with the facial injury; and a third surgery to attach the donor face to the recipient. Incisions and stitching would be made around the hairline and in the natural folds of the neck, and microsurgery techniques would be used to reattach the severed veins, arteries, and nerves necessary for tissue survival and muscular function (Wilson 2003). According to the surgeons, facial transplantation is technically easier than current approaches to facial reconstruction and involves considerably fewer surgeries.

## THE DONORS

At the time of writing, a number of severely disfigured persons have volunteered for the controversial surgery. The potential recipients and the surgical teams now anxiously await the world's first face donors. The question is: Who will these donors be?

With the recent publicity surrounding facial transplantation, some people may expressly choose to become face donors. While this is certainly a possibility, a more likely pool of candidates will be brain-dead patients who have signed an organ donor card that does not explicitly prohibit facial transplantation. At present, that would be most signed organ donor cards. Once these potential donors are identified, consistent with current practice for solid organ donation, family members presumably would be asked to consent to the removal of their loved one's face.

For all sorts of reasons, it is anticipated that there will be considerable difficulty in persuading families to consent to cadaveric face donation, even if they are willing to consent to cadaveric solid organ donation. In part, this will be difficult because the usual motivating factor—"giving the gift of life"—does not apply. Unlike solid organ transplantation, face transplantation is not a potentially life-saving intervention and so the face is not an organ that can easily be relabeled as a "gift of life." With facial transplantation, there is no underlying life-threatening condition; rather, the risk of death comes with the decision to proceed with the facial transplant in pursuit of improved quality of life.

Second, while families who consent to solid organ donation are often comforted by the thought that their loved one "lives on," it is not clear these same families want their kin to live on as someone else's face. After all, this doesn't fit well with the dominant transplant narrative that relies on the faceless category of the anonymous dead donor with reusable body parts (Sharp 2001). More generally, the face has tremendous symbolic and emotional value, and most surviving kin would not want to meet any resemblance of their dead relatives walking down the street. While computer modeling suggests that the recipients will not look like the donors (especially if the transplant does not include facial muscle, but is limited to skin that will be draped over a different bone structure), this concern may persist precisely because the face is personal in ways that other organs are not.

A final reason to expect limited enthusiasm for cadaveric face donation is that there is something rather ghoulish about agreeing to the removal of a loved one's face so that it can be gifted to someone else. One can't help but be reminded of numerous Hollywood B-movie horror plots that involve variations on the theme of stolen human body parts—facial or otherwise.

In addition to these personal challenges with organ donation, facial transplantation could potentially introduce social challenges to the existing organ retrieval system. Currently, there is a shortfall of donated organs and thousands of people remain on waiting lists (Veatch 2000). It is conceivable that this controversial practice could have a negative impact on the current system, should fewer people sign their organ donor cards for fear of losing their face. One solution to this problem might be to have organ-specific opting-out clauses that would allow prospective donors to specify that the face was not among the donated organs and tissues. For some, however, this might not provide sufficient assurances; even the remote possibility that, in error, the face would be removed would have them think twice about the whole organ donation process.

A second challenge to the current organ retrieval system might be renewed interest in controversial policies aimed at increasing the pool of organ donors, including decisions to offer burial fees and tax exemptions as donation incentives (Sharp 2001). Also, in recent years, a number of proposals have been developed supporting the buying and selling of organs. One such proposal would allow people to prospectively sell their organs. At the time of death, their organs would be removed and a prearranged sum would be paid to their estate. This procurement strategy, or a version thereof, might be promoted as a way of encouraging individuals to expressly choose face donation. This, and similar initiatives, could undermine the current system.

## THE RECIPIENTS

The primary benefit of facial transplantation for the recipient is improved quality of life through improved self-image and self-esteem and increased social interaction. To varying degrees, people with severe facial disfigurements (especially disfigured women) experience dysphoria, social anxiety, social phobia, and, less commonly, depression (Newell 2000, 386). With facial transplantation, the recipient will have one smooth skin surface, instead of a patchwork of skin with scar tissue and adhesions, and will experience some measure of restoration of facial expression and sensory function. Although the recipient's facial animation would likely still be quite restricted, for some this may compare favorably with conventional reconstructive surgeries, where the results are often less than satisfactory from both a cosmetic and a functional perspective. For example, with autologous transplantation, not only is the transplanted nonfacial skin typically not a good match, but often there is scar tissue and adhesions that affect appearance and restrict the use of facial muscles. The promise of facial transplantation is a "normal" appearance and nearly "normal" function (Wiggins et al. 2004). It is expected that these direct benefits will result in additional indirect benefits, including reduced social isolation, depression, and risk of suicide.

A key question in traditional bioethics is whether this potential benefit outweighs the potential harms. The most significant potential physical harms with facial transplantation are those associated with the surgery, the lifelong use of immunosuppressive drugs, and the risk of immune rejection. The surgical harms with facial transplantation are analogous to those with conventional reconstructive surgeries and include the possibility of a surgery nick or bruise to cranial nerves, which could result in limited muscular function or paralysis (and thus a limited range of expression).

Second, in addition to these potential surgical harms, there are the potential harms associated with the immunosuppression regimen. To reduce the risk of tissue rejection following transplantation, lifelong immunosuppression is prescribed. The long-term harms associated with this drug regimen are significant and include organ damage (e.g., kidney failure), cancer, diabetes, high blood pressure, and, in some instances, premature death. With facial transplantation, these harms, and in particular the risk of death, weigh heavily against the potential benefit of improved quality of life. Indeed, many have argued that while the risks of immunosuppressive therapy are worth taking when the alternative is death from a life-threatening condition that may be treated successfully with solid organ transplantation, these same risks are not worth taking with facial transplantation.

Third, despite the use of immune suppression drugs, there is still the risk of immune rejection. The 2003 Royal College report suggests a 10 percent chance of immediate rejection of the transplanted tissue (within six weeks), and a likely 30–50 percent chance of chronic rejection over a two- to five-year period (Royal College of Surgeons 2003). If the transplanted tissue is re-jected, it would have to be removed and replaced. If a suitable donor for a second facial transplant could not be identified, then conventional surgeries would have to be used to reconstruct a face using skin grafts and tissue flaps from other parts of the patients' own body, or engineered tissues.

Further, immune rejection may be a direct consequence of an inability or unwillingness to follow the immunosuppression regimen or to make the re-quired lifestyle changes in diet and sun exposure. For example, some people may be unable to tolerate the side effects of the prescribed drugs and may stop taking them. Clint Hallam, the first-hand transplant recipient, did not tolerate the immunosuppressive drugs. Eventually he stopped taking the drugs, the tissue began to deteriorate, and the hand had to be removed. It is conceivable that a face transplant recipient might have similar problems with the medications, in which case there might be similar consequences.

In addition to these potential physical harms, there are anticipated psy-chological harms. As summarized in the report of the Royal College of Sur-geons, these include:

> Fears relating to the viability of the transplanted organ; fear of the aftermath of possible rejection; anxiety relating to the potential side effects of immunosup-pressive medication, including increased risk of infection and malignancy; feel-ings of personal responsibility for the success or failure of the graft, linked to the need to adhere to a drug regimen, the need to alter some behaviour patterns such as diet and sun exposure, the monitoring of symptoms, and regular atten-dance at numerous out-patient appointments; integration of the transplant into an existing body image and sense of identity; and emotional responses to the ex-perience of receiving a transplanted organ, including feelings of gratitude and guilt in relation to the donor and the donor's family. (2003, 9)

Of these possible harms, "integration of the transplant into an existing body image and sense of identity" is of particular concern. For people with a seri-ous facial disfigurement, body image and sense of identity may already be a source of considerable emotional distress and social problems.

All told, though considerable uncertainty remains, for some persons with serious facial anomalies, the anticipated benefits of facial transplantation are believed to outweigh the potential harms, and they are prepared to consent to the proposed surgery.

## THE RESEARCH

In very general terms, for consent by a competent person to be a morally valid choice, there typically needs to be full disclosure, adequate under-standing, freedom from coercion, and authorization (Faden and Beauchamp 1986).

As regards the need for full disclosure, it is imperative that prospective transplant recipients know that the proposed surgical intervention is not a therapeutic intervention "designed solely to enhance the well-being of an individual patient or client" (Levine 1988, 3–4). At best, face transplantation, like other experimental surgeries, is a nonvalidated practice; reliable data about safety and efficacy are lacking, as is professional consensus about the therapeutic merits of the surgery. For this nonvalidated practice to become standard practice, it must first be validated through research that aims to develop or contribute to generalizable knowledge. It is important to emphasize this point about the nature of facial transplantation, because transplant surgeons willingly describe the surgery as an innovative therapeutic procedure (Wiggins et al. 2004) and describe themselves as clinicians (Butler, Clarke, and Ashcroft 2004). These descriptions are deeply problematic because they foster a therapeutic misconception: the potential face recipient needs to know that facial transplantation is ultimately about research, not therapy. This is not to deny the general hope that the patient will benefit from the surgery. It is to recognize properly, however, that the primary objective is not to enhance patient well-being by providing a safe and effective therapy, but rather to generate and validate new knowledge.

In addition to providing information about the nature of the proposed transplant, it is imperative that the surgeons address the issue of false hopes and expectations that may be associated with technical success. The hope with facial transplantation is that it will restore appearance and mobility. Instead of a patchwork of skin grafts and tissue flaps, there will be a smooth surface; instead of a masklike face, there will be "acceptable" reanimation; instead of rejection, there will be social integration; instead of loneliness, there will be love. In sum, "fix my face, fix my life, my soul" (Grealy 1994, 215). The hopes of those who have suffered a serious facial trauma may be unrealistic. Even if the surgery is technically successful (meaning the tissue is not rejected and there is between 50 and 70 percent reanimation in a year or so), the transplant recipient may be looking for a "new" life through some form of personal and social transformation, and this just may not happen.

Next, in considering the issue of voluntariness, it is important to remember that, by definition, consent is always revocable up until such time as the consented-to intervention has been undertaken, at which point the option of withdrawal is moot (except in a research context, where there may still be the option of withdrawing one's data from the aggregated research findings). Research consent forms typically include a clause that reminds the research participant of her right to withdraw from research without fear of consequences, such as limited access to care.

Face transplant recipients, like all research participants, retain the right to withdraw from research. A decision to withdraw from facial transplantation research post transplant may be particularly difficult to manage, however. For example, the recipient may choose to withdraw from the research by refusing to continue with the required immunosuppressive regimen because of difficulties tolerating the drugs, because of the high costs of the medications (Sharp 1999), because of dissatisfaction with the outcome, because of psychological problems adjusting to the new face, or simply because she has a death wish. Should the recipient so decide, the transplant team would be faced with an interesting challenge, if we presume an a priori commitment to respecting patient autonomy. If the recipient stops taking her medications, tissue rejection will follow. If she then will not consent to further autologous transplantation, transplantation using genetically engineered tissue cultures, or a facial prosthesis, death will follow. Do the transplant surgeons simply accept the recipient's withdrawal from research as an exercise of free choice? Or, is apparent respect for patient autonomy in this case a form of abandonment? What are the transplant surgeons' moral obligations given this possible denouement? Does one simply stand by and witness what might be described as an unusual form of suicide?

In addition to the right to withdraw, there is also the right to privacy and confidentiality. In the abstract, this shouldn't be an issue with facial transplantation. There is considerable experience with anonymous solid organ donation, and a huge infrastructure is in place to protect the anonymity of donors and recipients. But anonymity doesn't appear to be part of the plan, and this is in some measure because of the way in which reporting science changed in the late 1970s with the birth of the world's first test-tube baby, Louise Brown, and in the early 1980s with the Jarvik-7 artificial heart for Barney Clark. These events marked an important shift away from reporting major medical and scientific advances in peer-reviewed professional journals, to reporting "high-profile human-interest research" in press releases with grand announcements of "first-in-the-world" breakthroughs. The reasons typically given for this shift are the public's "right to know" and "freedom of the press" (Morreim 2004). But the more mundane truth is that the shift to press releases and frequent media updates with patient-specific information is more about the thrill of sleuthing on the part of reporters, increased sales on the part of media outlets, self-aggrandizement on the part of researchers and their institutions, advertisement under the guise of news, and voyeurism on our part.

While it may not be possible in a contemporary context to promise privacy and confidentiality, there is quite a difference between issuing press releases that promote media interest and making concerted efforts to minimize the risk of media intrusion. Failure to commit to trying to protect privacy and confidentiality speaks to another ethical issue—conflict of interest. Of late, discussions concerning conflict of interest in research typically focus on financial conflicts, and the remedy invariably proposed is full disclosure. This is not the concern alluded to here, though there may be financial rewards for those participating in the surgery. The possible conflict of concern is that which exists between the career interests of members of the surgical teams and the best interests of the research participants. In response to this possible conflict, some surgeons will object that respect for privacy and confidentiality conflicts with the interests of science, not personal interests. In their view, privacy and confidentiality cannot be guaranteed because of the need to include unaltered photographs of the facial transplant in professional peer-reviewed publications. Perhaps, but how does this explain or justify press releases? This is surely no way to go about dimming "the intense media spotlight" (Wiggins et al. 2004).

## ETRE BIEN DANS SA PEAU

There is an expression in French, "Etre bien dans sa peau," for which I have never been able to offer an adequate translation. A literal translation is "to be well in one's skin"; a nuanced interpretation is "to be comfortable with oneself." The beauty of the French expression is that it captures both of these discrete ideas in the one classic phrase—a phrase that identifies the importance of being at ease with oneself, while explicitly recognizing, through reference to the skin, the embodied (corporeal) nature of that self. Self and sense of self are key issues with facial transplantation. The face—our most intimate and individual characteristic—is critical to our sense of who we are. This is no less true for persons with unusual faces. James Partridge, a burn victim, reminds us, "Even for those like myself with severe disfigurement, the face carries a lot of identity, the sense of self" (McDowell 2002).

Elsewhere I have argued that selfhood is a dynamic process that is both fostered and challenged by the world in which we live and the stories that we are able to construct and maintain. In this view, who we are is inexorably shaped by personal and environmental factors. The personal factors include individual attributes (e.g., an unusual face) and personal life experiences (e.g., serious trauma to the face that results in permanent disfigurement). The environmental factors include all others with whom we engage, in the context of either close interpersonal relations or other relations of mutual recognition. Our intimate and distant interactions with others influence how we see ourselves, which in turn influences how we act and interact in the world, which in turn influences how others see and interact with us, which in turn influences how we see ourselves. In this way, our interactions with others both shape and stabilize our sense of self over time. These interactions and their mutually reinforcing influences establish our narrative identity—an identity constructed for and by the self through stories "acquired, refined, revised, displaced, and replaced" over time through introspection and continued lived experience (Baylis 2003, 145). It is through our stories that we make sense of our place in the world—where we are from, where we have been, and where we are going.

Our face, be it our original face, our disfigured face, our mended face, or our transplanted face, is of central importance in our stories. For just as our stories help us to make sense of where we are from and where we are going, so too our face helps "us understand who we are and where we come from. . . . [It follows that a] disruption to one's facial appearance, especially the inability to recognize oneself, represents a profound disruption of body image and may constitute a major life crisis" (Royal College of Surgeons 2003, 9). Notably, the disruption can occur not only at the time of injury but also following reconstructive surgery, and possibly again following facial transplantation.

A key insight with narrative identity is that both internal and external factors are relevant to the construction of self. "We are both who we say we are (based on our own interpretation and reconstruction of personal stories), and who others will let us be (as mediated through historical, social, cultural, political, religious and other contexts)" (Baylis 2003, 148–49). For this reason, a traumatic facial injury resulting in permanent disfigurement will have a significant impact on "the ongoing process of identity formation—which involves a complex interaction between 'self'-perception, 'self'-projection, 'other'-perception and 'other'-reaction" (149). The impact will be in terms of cosmetic appearance and ability to communicate.

We live in an extremely visual world with a relatively narrow (some might say shallow) sense of what is attractive. Indeed, from a young age, children notice disfigurement and learn to prefer attractive to unattractive people. With increasing age, this prejudice often extends to a preference for persons who have no disabilities (Newell 2000, 386). In this world, facially disfigured people experience verbal abuse, disgust, and pity—and so, not surprisingly, they experience psychological distress and social problems.

A serious facial injury, treated by conventional means, typically results in an unusual face. This new face is generally threatening to the self, as it disrupts intimate personal relations as well as distant relations of mutual recognition. As one burn victim, Gwedolyn Arrington, explains, she cannot go out in public without attracting open uncensored stares: "Little toddlers might say: 'Look at the monster.' Or, people just walk into walls. . . . Most people have the benefit of blending in. I don't have that option when I go outside" (Taylor 2004). "All I really want is to walk down the street and not be so noticeable" (Weiss 2004). Within her family there were also personal hurts that were just as severe, as when her two-year-old daughter "was initially repulsed by her appearance" (Taylor 2004).

Lucy Grealy, a woman with a facial disfigurement following surgery for cancer, muses: "What would it be like to walk down the street and be able to trust that no one would say anything nasty to me? My only clues were from Halloween and from the winter, when I could wrap up the lower half of my face in a scarf. . . . To feel that confidence without the threat of exposure—how could I possibly want anything more?" (Grealy 1994, 157) If one accepts that "identity formation is an ongoing process of self-construction influenced by personal attributes, life experiences, introspection, and the storying

of one's life" (Baylis 2004, 31), then threats to personal and other social relations resulting from facial disfigurement are significant threats to personal
identity.

Second, serious facial disfigurements typically alter one's ability to communicate effectively. Two-thirds of our communications are facial, and this
nonverbal communication is critical to establishing and maintaining successful relationships (Royal College of Surgeons 2003, 10). Without words,
through both conscious and unconscious facial expressions, our families,
friends, colleagues, and even strangers can read expressions of sadness, per-
plexity, confusion, and joy on our faces. When these expressions are absent,
or distorted, miscommunication is common and this contributes to difficulties with social interaction.


## THE SELF IN THE SHADOW OF THE "SELF"

To state the obvious, a facial transplant could have as profound an impact on
identity as the original facial trauma. The surgery will introduce significant
changes in appearance and affect one's patterns of communication. Let us
imagine a technically successful facial transplantation where all outward
signs of lived trauma are erased and social interaction is not hindered by appearance or communication difficulties (albeit at the cost of lifelong immunosuppression and all of the attendant risks). Even with this best-case
scenario, however, identity issues will be of concern because of the cultural
meaning (and reading) of faces.

Past experience with organ transplantation suggests that face recipients
may have an altered sense of embodiment following the surgery. According
to Margaret Lock, "Donated organs very often represent much more than
mere biological body parts; the life with which they are animated is experienced by recipients as personified, an agency that manifests itself in some
surprising ways and profoundly influences subjectivity" (2002, 1409). Some
solid organ recipients experience new eating habits and new recreational interests. They assume that these foreign experiences belong to the donor. This
has lead to questions about the possibility of somatic (or body) memory.
Now consider face transplantation: If there is such a thing as somatic memory, what would it mean for the transplant recipient to not only fail to recognize herself in the mirror, but also to fail to recognize certain experiences
as her own? (Baylis 2004, 31). As a result, might the new face be psychologically rejected as "foreign," or as "other"?

Gwedolyn Arrington says, "I know there will be some psychological adjustments because it's not your own skin. . . . But, in terms of not looking like
myself, I already feel that way. I don't look like myself: I wasn't born like
this. So, I don't even see myself when I look in the mirror now" (Taylor

2004). "With all the grafts I've received, patches here and patches there, I honestly feel like I'm already living with someone else's face" (Weiss 2004). Exchanging one strange face for another, however, may still result in significant emotional distress, especially if the anticipated improvements in quality of life are not forthcoming. More generally, it is impossible to predict whether adjusting to wearing someone else's face will be any easier than adjusting to one's own disfigured face.

Whatever the personal experience, there will be a complex renegotiation of the self in the broader social context, where family and friends will have to adjust to a new facial appearance and changes in nonverbal communication. If the response of others to these changes is discordant with the recipient's expectations, there will be difficulty in reconstructing one's identity and stabilizing the hoped-for self. This instability risks calling forward the transplant recipient's doppelgänger and relegating the authentic self to the shadows.

The well-known concept of the doppelgänger (literally double-self) appears in Lucy Grealy's autobiography when she writes of her own experience following years of grafts and revision operations to her face:

> I didn't look like me. . . . I couldn't make what I saw in the mirror correspond to the person I thought I was. It wasn't only that I continued to feel ugly; I simply could not conceive of the image as belonging to me. . . . I felt I was being mistaken for someone else. The person in the mirror was an imposter—why couldn't anyone else see this? (1994, 219)

A potential problem for the recipient of a successful facial transplant is that the person visible to family and friends may not be the true self. How so? A successful facial transplant can remove the scarred tissue and thereby mask a once-visible social biography. The transplant, however, cannot remove the scarred person or disembody that social biography. At most, the transplant can disguise some of the evidence of serious trauma to the face by removing the mask that is this patchwork of skin and replacing it with another mask that hides the traumatized self—the person with emotional scars that are an integral part of who she is. This is not an argument against facial transplantation, but rather a call for increased awareness of the incredible complexity of identity formation. In the final analysis, a technically successful facial transplantation may still result in a failure of lived experience, as when the recipient painfully perceives that someone other than herself, an interloper no less, is the protagonist in her public life, her social world.

### NOTE

Sincere thanks are owed to Lynette Reid and David Benatar for helpful comments on an earlier draft and to Michael Bolton for editorial assistance.

# REFERENCES

Baylis, Françoise. 2003. Black as me: Narrative identity. *Developing World Bioethics* 3 (2): 142–50.
———. 2004. A face is not just like a hand: *Pace* Barker. *American Journal of Bioethics* 4 (3): 30–32.
BBC. 1998. From hand to face. BBC News, September 30. Available at http://news.bbc.co.uk/1/hi/health/183870.stm.
Butler, Peter, Alex Clarke, and Richard Ashcroft. 2004. Face transplantation: When and for whom? *American Journal of Bioethics* 4 (3): 16–17.
CBS. 2004. Clinic gets OK on face transplants. CBS News, November 1. Available at http://www.cbsnews.com/stories/2004/09/17/health/main644116.shtml.
CCNE. 2004. Composite tissue allotransplantation (CTA) of the face (full or partial facial transplant). Opinion No. 082. National Consultative Bioethics Committee for Health and Life Sciences, Paris, France, February 6. Available at http://www.ccne-ethique.fr.
Cleveland Clinic Foundation. 2004. Cleveland Clinic approves patient protocol for facial tissue transplantation. Press release, November 4.
Dougherty, Hugh. 2003. Burns girl to have first face transplant. *Evening Standard*. February 28. Available at http://www.thisislondon.com/news/articles/3609267?
Dubernard, Jean-Michel, Earl Owen, Guillaume Herzberg, Marco Lanzetta, Xavier Martin, Hari Kapila, Marwan Dawahara, and Nadley S Hakim. 1999. Human hand allograft: Report on first 6 months. *Lancet* 353: 1315–20.
Dubernard, Jean-Michel, Earl Owen, Nicole LeFrancois, Palmina Petruzzo, Xavier Martin, Marwan Dawahra, Denis Jullien, Jean Kanitakis, Camille Frances, Xavier Preville, Lucette Gebuhrer, Nadey Hakim, Marco Lanzetta, Hary Kapila, Guillaume Herzberg, and Jean-Pierre Revillard. 2000. First human hand transplant: Case report. *Transplant International* 13, suppl. 1: S521–S524.
Faden, Ruth, and Tom Beauchamp. 1986. *A history and theory of consent*. New York: Oxford University Press.
Grealy, Lucy. 1994. *Autobiography of a face*. New York: Harper Perennial.
Hettiaratchy, Shehan, and Peter Butler. 2003. Extending the boundaries of transplantation: Recent hand transplants may herald a new era. *British Medical Journal* 326: 1226–27.
Levine, Robert. *Ethics and regulation of clinical research*. 2nd ed. New Haven: Yale University Press, 1988. [These definitions are based on those first articulated in: National Commission, "The Belmont Report: Ethical Principles and Guidelines for the Protection of Human Subjects of Research," DHEW Pub. No. (OS) 78-0012 (1978), 2–4.]
Lock, Margaret. 2002. Human body parts as therapeutic tools: Contradictory discourses and transformed subjectivities. *Qualitative Health Research* 12 (10): 1406–18.
McDowell, Natasha. 2002. Surgeons struggle with ethical nightmare of face transplants. *Nature* 420: 449.
Morreim, Haavi. 2004. High-profile research and the media: The case of the AbioCor Artificial Heart. *Hastings Center Report* 34 (1): 11–24.
Newell, R. 2000. Psychological difficulties amongst plastic surgery ex-patients following surgery to the face: A survey. *British Journal of Plastic Surgery* 53: 386–92.
Royal College of Surgeons [Royal College of Surgeons of England Working Party: P. Morris, A. Bradley, L. Doyal, M. Earley, M. Milling, and N. Rumsey]. 2003. *Facial Transplantation: Working Party Report*. November. Available at http://www.rcseng.ac.uk/publications/docs/facial_transplantation.html/view?searchterm=Facial%20Transplantation.
Sharp, Lesley A. 1999. A medical anthropologist's view on posttransplant compliance. The underground economy of medical survival. *Transplantation Proceedings* 31, suppl. 4A: 31S–33S.
———. 2001. Commodified kin: Death, mourning, and competing claims on the bodies of organ donors in the United States. *American Anthropologist* 103 (1): 112–33.

Taylor, Paul. 2004. Face transplants: Dead men walking? *Globe and Mail*, 17 December.
Veatch, Robert. 2000. *Transplantation ethics*. Washington, DC: Georgetown University Press.
Weiss, Rick. 2004. Face transplants raise hopes—and some fears. *Washington Post*, November 8. Available at http://www.washingtonpost.com/ac2/wp-dyn/A32875-2004Nov7?
Wiggins, Osborne, John Barker, Serge Martinez, Marieke Vossen, Claudio Maldonado, Federico V. Grossi, Cedric G. Francoise, Michael Cunningham, Gustavo Perez-Abadia, Moshe Kon, and Joseph C. Banis. 2004. On the ethics of facial transplantation research. *American Journal of Bioethics* 4 (3): 1–12.
Wilson, Jim. 2003. Trading faces. *Popular Mechanics* 180 (11): 77.

# V

# COSMETIC SURGERY

A Defense of Cosmetic Surgery
*Stephen Coleman*

Beauty under the Knife: A Feminist Appraisal of Cosmetic Surgery
*Rosemarie Tong and Hilde Lindemann*

# 10

✛

# A Defense
# of Cosmetic Surgery

*Stephen Coleman*

The practice of cosmetic surgery has been criticized since its inception around the end of the 19th century. Many early cosmetic surgeons were derided as "quacks," as untrained charlatans, or as tricksters who only desired to make a fast buck at the expense of vain or silly women who were overly preoccupied with their appearance. Such surgeons were often seen as being outside the boundaries of the medical establishment or as engaged in practices that were not properly classified as a form of medicine at all. Some of these criticisms, perhaps even all of them, continue to the present day. In this chapter I wish to attempt to defend what many still see as indefensible, the practice of cosmetic surgery.

I should begin by making it clear what I am actually attempting to defend. Cosmetic surgery is one branch of the medical specialty of plastic surgery, which also includes such things as reconstructive surgery. Here, when I use the term *cosmetic surgery*, I specifically want to exclude reconstructive surgery from the definition. Thus for the purposes of this chapter, I will define *cosmetic surgery* as surgery undertaken to alter a person's appearance (usually from its natural state) for reasons other than a response to injury, disease, or genetic or other disorder. This does not accord with everyday uses of the terms "plastic surgery" or "cosmetic surgery," which are generall' used interchangeably in the popular press (such as in "Hollywood Star Amazing $40,000 Plastic Surgery" or "Disfigured Fijian Boy's Incredi' Cosmetic Surgery Transformation"). My concern here is solely to defend practice of cosmetic surgery (also known at times as "aesthetic surger' "vanity surgery") and not the far more acceptable reconstructive aspe plastic surgery. When it is necessary to refer to other forms of plastic s in this chapter, I will use the term *plastic surgery* to refer to the full '

practices within the specialty and *reconstructive surgery* to refer to surgery undertaken to modify a person's appearance in response (at least partially) to injury, disease, or genetic disorder.

The discussion that follows proceeds in two main sections. In the first, I will discuss the distinction between reconstructive surgery and cosmetic surgery, in an attempt to show that what might intuitively seem to be a clear distinction is in fact far hazier than is usually acknowledged. The overall aim of this section is to try to get a firm(ish) grasp of what cosmetic surgery is, so as to make it clear exactly what I will need to defend. In the second section, I will discuss the ways in which the concept of autonomy might impact on the practice of cosmetic surgery, and how this concept might provide a general defense of this particular branch of medicine.

## RECONSTRUCTIVE SURGERY MEETS COSMETIC SURGERY

Few people have ever expressed concerns about the reconstructive aspects of plastic surgery, and this aspect of plastic surgery is seen as an appropriate function of medical intervention. Reconstruction of bodies and faces ravaged by fire, disease, or genetic conditions are both reasonably common and the subject of the plaudits of society when such surgeries come under the public gaze. In fact it was in the aftermath of World War I that plastic surgery first came to achieve respectability, in the treatment of returned soldiers whose bodily features had been deformed by the effects of shrapnel, gas, and other machinery of war.

Reconstructive surgery, unlike cosmetic surgery, is also usually available under publicly funded medical programs, and it is this aspect upon which I wish to focus my discussion for a moment. Medical services that are not seen as a necessity for patient health and well-being, those that might be deemed as frivolous, nonessential, elective, or "luxury" services, will not be funded by the public purse. The fact that reconstructive surgery *is* available through government funding gives some indication of the acceptability of the practice and is a very strong indication that this sort of medical intervention is seen by those in government and in the medical profession as a necessity for patient health and well-being.

I must make mention at this point of the commonly discussed (and disputed) treatment/enhancement distinction. One of the ways in which this distinction is employed is to suggest that only those forms of medicine on the treatment side of the divide ought to be publicly funded, and that any form of medical intervention that aims at enhancement rather than treatment ought not to receive any form of public funding. The space constraints of this discussion do not allow any real discussion of this issue here, other than to note that given such a distinction, it could be argued that any form of plastic surgery that has been deemed eligible for public funding ought to

be seen as a form of treatment, rather than as a form of enhancement. Another, rather more controversial, use of the treatment/enhancement distinction is the suggestion that the aim of medicine ought to be treatment, and not enhancement. If such a distinction can be justified, and if the practice of cosmetic surgery is to be defended as a legitimate aim of medicine, then it would need to find a home on the treatment side of the equation.

With these ideas in mind, I wish to consider the health care situation in the Netherlands, where plastic surgery was, for a time, included in the basic health care package.[1] Any individual who could demonstrate that he or she required plastic surgery was entitled to have the surgery paid for by national health insurance. When this national health insurance scheme came under increasing financial pressure and those administering the scheme had to decide where to scale it back, they decided to remove cosmetic surgery from the scheme, while still including reconstructive surgery. The difficulties that were experienced in drawing such a line illustrate the problems that one faces in attempting to determine exactly what procedures might qualify as cosmetic, rather than reconstructive, surgery.

After considerable debate, a committee, comprising representatives of medicine and the national heath insurance companies, established categories of plastic surgery that were deemed "necessary" and would thus continue to be funded by the public purse. In establishing these categories, the committee was attempting to differentiate between what they called "medically necessary" cosmetic surgery (by my definitions a form of reconstructive surgery) and nonessential elective or "luxury" cosmetic surgery. One category of "medically necessary" cosmetic surgery, which caused very little difficulty, was plastic surgery for patients whose appearance had been disfigured or deformed through accident, injury, or disease. The remaining, more controversial, categories covered procedures for patients who wished to have plastic surgery to alter their appearance from its original "natural" form; that is, for patients whose appearance—though not altered through accident, injury, or disease—was still felt to warrant medical intervention. The three categories that were introduced were:

1. A functional disturbance or affliction (e.g., eyelids that droop to such an extent that vision is impaired).
2. Severe psychological suffering (the patient is under psychiatric treatment specifically for problems with appearance).
3. A physical imperfection that falls "outside a normal degree of variation in appearance."

It was the third category that proved to be most difficult to deal with, since the committee had to create some standards to define exactly what fell "outside a normal degree of variation in appearance," and these standards had to be set for each individual cosmetic surgery procedure. Thus it was that prospective

patients for a breast lift had to show that their nipples were level with their el-
bows, and prospective liposuction recipients had to demonstrate a difference in
four clothing sizes between the top and bottom halves of their bodies. Prospective face-lift patients had to prove that their face made them appear to be ten
years older than their chronological age, and patients seeking eyelid corrections
had to prove that they looked like they had been out drinking all evening (presumably without actually going out and drinking all evening!).

Some types of procedure were simply excluded altogether. An example of
this sort was tattoo removal. The argument was that, since the tattoos had
been applied voluntarily at one's own expense, they ought to be removed in
the same way. This was, theoretically, a textbook example of a purely cosmetic procedure. But problems arose when many Moroccan immigrant
women applied to have tattoos removed. While tattooing may be considered
voluntary in the Netherlands, women in Morocco were commonly tattooed
under coercion as a symbol of cultural constraint. The removal of such tattoos thus came to be seen as a form of reconstructive surgery, necessary for
the integration of these migrant women into Dutch society, and thus necessary for the well-being of these women. Given that this form of tattoo
removal was a type of reconstructive surgery, it was accepted that tattoo
removal should be paid for by the national health insurance, provided that
the patient was female and not Dutch born.

Of course, it was not long after this decision was made that another case
arose which caused the authorities to again broaden the definition of reconstructive surgery. A Dutch-born woman applied for tattoo removal and was
duly denied coverage under the rules of the national health insurance. But
when the facts of the case became public—it was revealed that this woman
had been drugged and raped, after which her assailant had tattooed his
name onto her stomach—this ruling was revised. Again this form of plastic
surgery was deemed to be reconstructive rather than simply cosmetic. The
procedure for removing tattoos had been excluded from the Dutch national
health insurance coverage on the grounds that it did not seem to fall into any
of the three categories, though in cases like the ones above it was felt that the
tattoos were causing severe psychological distress, and thus it was reasonable for the public purse to pay for their removal.

Even more problematic than this were questions about what procedures,
and more important what particular cases, ought to be included in the third
category. After several years of argument about this issue, a decision was finally made to remove the third criterion of surgery entirely from the national
health insurance scheme, so that variation in appearance that fell outside the
normal range would no longer be accepted as a criterion for state-funded
plastic surgery. Surgery indicated by functional disturbance or severe psychological distress would still receive public funding.

Despite the fact that the public purse was supposed to fund plastic surgery
that was necessary to alleviate severe psychological distress for the patient, in

fact requests for payment for surgery under this criterion have generally been refused, usually for one of two reasons. Either it was felt that the problem was not severe enough to warrant surgery ("who doesn't have some problem with their appearance?") or it was felt that the problems for the patient were deemed to be too severe ("this patient has so much wrong with them that a mere nip and tuck isn't going to make any difference"). In fact, for at least some patients who appealed the decision that had been passed against them, both reasons were given, one in the initial decision, and the other in the refusal-of-payment decision given against the patient upon appeal.

While this discussion might appear to be little more than an amusing sideline, it does have a serious purpose. My aim in this chapter is to defend cosmetic surgery, which I defined as surgery undertaken to alter a person's appearance but not in response to injury, disease, or genetic or other disorder. I hope that this discussion has shown that many types of plastic surgery which may seem to have been undertaken purely for reasons of appearance are actually supported by other reasons. The removal of tattoos of immigrant women, for example, while certainly changing their appearance, was actually undertaken to allow these women to cast off the outward symbols of cultural oppression and to allow them to better integrate themselves into Dutch society. The removal of the tattoo from the rape victim was clearly going to be necessary if she was to have any realistic chance of recovery from the trauma of her assault. Procedures aimed at dealing with some particular facet of a person's appearance that is causing psychological problems are intended to treat those psychological problems, rather than being undertaken merely for reasons of appearance. Surgery to correct the droop of eyelids that interfere with vision is actually aimed at allowing the patient to achieve proper visual function, and so on.

In light of this, it is interesting to examine what is often seen as the paradigm case of pure cosmetic surgery: the Hollywood actress who seeks plastic surgery in an attempt to retain her youthful appearance. The specific example that I wish to consider comes from the June 14, 2004, issue of *Woman's Day*. This popular Australian women's magazine ran as its cover story a piece on Sharon Stone's (apparent) face-lift surgery, complete with before and after photos, expert comment on the procedures that had apparently been undertaken, comment on how much more attractive she looked after this expert surgery, estimates of the cost of the procedures,[2] and so on. Most interesting as far as this current discussion is concerned, however, was the short segment mentioning how much more in demand as an actress Stone would now be, and discussing the fact that virtually all "older" actresses are now forced to turn to plastic surgery at some stage if they wish to continue to find work. The article even implied that Stone had bucked the trend by putting off plastic surgery for so long, but that she had been forced to accept the necessity of plastic surgery after failing to gain any recent worthwhile movie roles.

I do not want to get into an argument about whether or not Sharon Stone has actually had plastic surgery, since I am much more interested in the issues raised in the article about the motivation for actresses like her to take such steps. If an actress such as Stone was to have this type of surgery, and if the surgery was motivated by her desire to continue working as an actress (and this does seem to be a reasonable suggestion under the circumstances), then I would suggest that face-lift surgery, such as she is alleged to have had, does not actually qualify as cosmetic surgery under my definition, since the surgery was not undertaken purely, or even primarily, for the purpose of appearance, but was rather undertaken as a means to an end, that of allowing her to resume her career as an actress. While we might well deride Hollywood for its sexist stance in this matter (since male stars certainly do not experience the same pressures to look youthful as female stars do), given the acknowledged fact that there are few, if any, worthwhile roles for older-looking women, it must be acknowledged that it is indeed *necessary* for most Hollywood actresses to seek plastic surgery in order to continue to work in their chosen field. This point is made explicitly in another magazine article on the subject of plastic surgery, where Anna Gauche, a Los Angeles–based cosmetic dermatologist, is quoted:

> There is a mad rush that begins at about age 40 to look 10 years younger. For actresses, their looks *are* their jobs. People come in saying they're losing auditions. It's not an issue of vanity. It's a necessity.[3]

A very similar argument can be mounted with regard to the breast augmentation surgery being sought by many much younger actresses. If it is true, other things being equal, that directors and casting agencies will offer roles to actresses with larger breasts over actresses with smaller breasts, then it can be argued that when a young actress seeks breast augmentation surgery, she is not doing so primarily for reasons of appearance but rather because that it is what is necessary for success in that field. If this is so, then this type of surgery would also not qualify as cosmetic surgery under my definition.

In fact, since the very early days of modern plastic surgery, it has been common for women to seek surgery not because they simply wanted to improve their appearance or to look younger, but because they felt that it was necessary. One of the first textbooks of cosmetic surgery, written in 1926 by the first famous female cosmetic surgeon, Madame Noël (credited as the pioneer of the face-lift), refers to "the bitter need" behind her female patient's desires to surgically improve their appearance.[4] This need to which she referred is purely economic; Noël provided a series of cases that illustrate the financial problems that older women faced in Paris in the first quarter of the twentieth century (when Noël was working and writing): the aging opera singer no longer asked to sing in spite of her beautiful voice, the seamstress unable to secure a supervisory position in the sweatshop, the experienced sales manager fired in favor of a younger woman, and so on. Noël suggests that none of these women would have sought her services were it not for their need to appear more youthful in order to retain, or to reclaim, employment. In none of these cases were the patients seeking merely to improve their looks; all of the cases mentioned by Madame Noël are cases where plastic surgery was sought due to necessity. Thus none of these cases fall under my definition of cosmetic surgery.

Many other pioneers of plastic surgery worked in specific ways in order to alleviate the particular problems of their patients, often problems with other people's perceptions of the patient's appearances. For example, the German surgeon Jacques Joseph, known in plastic surgery circles as the father of the nose correction, worked in the late 1920s and early 1930s in Germany. A large number of his nose job patients were Jews who sought surgery to reduce the size of their noses to "gentile proportions."[5] While these patients certainly wished to alter their appearances, it is clear that the surgery they sought was not undertaken simply to improve their appearance, but rather to help them to try to avoid the anti-Semitism that they faced. Surgery is still often sought to assist people in overcoming prejudices; particularly common is surgery to reduce the obviousness of stereotypical racial features, such as nose "corrections" to give blacks more "Anglo" noses, or eyelid surgery to give Asian eyes a more open appearance.[6] While the object of such surgery is certainly to change the patient's appearance, and while we might deplore the prejudices of a society that makes people feel that such surgery is necessary, again it is clear that the object of the surgery is to help these people avoid prejudice, rather than simply to alter their appearance. Again, such surgery does not meet my definition of cosmetic surgery.

Indeed, one might wonder whether *any* plastic surgery will meet my classification of cosmetic surgery; perhaps my definition simply defines an empty set. It may well be the case that no plastic surgery can be said to aim *merely* at changing the appearance of the patient, since the patient seeks this appearance-altering surgery for a particular reason. Flat-chested women seeking breast augmentation surgery, for example, often suggest that they are undergoing such surgery in order to feel more self-confident. Many other patients feel that they possess one particular feature that is abnormal and seek surgery not to make themselves attractive but to make themselves "normal."[7] Those who work in particular industries, particularly in entertainment or fashion, may seek surgery because they feel it is essential for success in that industry. None of these people seek surgery *purely* to improve their appearance, so none of these cases would meet my definition of cosmetic surgery.

If all cases of apparent cosmetic surgery involve reasons other than merely altering one's appearance, then it could be argued that cosmetic surgery, as I have defined it, does not exist. Thus a defense of these contested forms of plastic surgery would simply amount to demonstrating that such forms of surgery share key features with uncontested forms of plastic surgery and thus that what appears, on first glance, to be cosmetic surgery is actually a form of reconstructive surgery.

However, there are reasons why I do not wish to end the discussion at this point. For one thing, it doesn't really seem to be a satisfactory solution to a problem such as this to simply define the problem out of existence. More important, the argument that I have presented does not conclusively prove that cases of cosmetic surgery, as I have defined it, do not exist; rather it demonstrates that there is no way of clearly differentiating cases of reconstructive surgery from cases of cosmetic surgery. To make the move from (a) showing that there is no clear line between reconstructive surgery and cosmetic surgery to (b) claiming that cosmetic surgery does not exist, is no more plausible than moving from (x) showing that there is no clear line between hairiness and baldness to (y) claiming that baldness does not exist.[8] While it might well be the case that cosmetic surgery, as I have defined it, does not exist, one cannot reach such a conclusion from the fact that there is no clear distinction between reconstructive and cosmetic surgery, although one can certainly argue (as I have done) that there are actually fewer cases of cosmetic surgery, and more cases of reconstructive surgery, than might appear on first glance.

I will thus assume that at least some cases of cosmetic surgery, as I have defined it, *do* exist, and I will attempt to defend this practice of cosmetic surgery with reference to the concept of individual autonomy, trusting that such a defense would also be sufficient for other types of plastic surgery that, while not meeting my strict definition of cosmetic surgery, might also seem to some to require some justification.

## AUTONOMY AND COSMETIC SURGERY

In order to contain this discussion to a reasonable length, I will be forced to make some assumptions about personal autonomy. I will, without argument, define autonomy as "being able to understand and act upon one's considered values and commitments."[9] I will also assume that personal autonomy is an important value within society and that moral agents within society have what amounts to a right to exercise their autonomy, as long as this exercise of autonomy does not interfere with the autonomy of others or cause harm to other moral beings. I recognize that such assumptions may not meet with universal approval, but I do think (and hope) that such views meet with sufficient approval that I can proceed to the heart of my defense of cosmetic surgery without providing any defense for these assumptions.

If moral agents possess a right to exercise their autonomy, then this would generally allow those agents to seek out and obtain cosmetic surgery, if such surgery acts as an expression of, or assists in the expression of, that agent's considered values and commitments. After all, the exercise of autonomy is considered sufficient reason to allow moral agents to modify their bodies in other, more or less permanent ways, such as through the acquisition of such things as tattoos and body piercings. It would seem strange indeed if the exercise of autonomy was seen as sufficient justification for these sorts of permanent bodily changes but insufficient for a person to modify his or her body in more or less permanent ways through the application of cosmetic surgery. In order to make that argument—that the exercise of autonomy is not sufficient justification for seeking cosmetic surgery while it is for acquiring other permanent bodily changes such as tattoos—one would need to make the case that there is some morally significant difference between tattooing and cosmetic surgery.

I can see two ways in which such an argument might be mounted. One would be to argue that cosmetic surgery carries much greater risks to one's health than tattooing or body piercing. While this makes no real difference to the person seeking cosmetic surgery (since respect for autonomy requires us to respect the fact that others may not evaluate risk and reward in the same way we do), it does highlight one important issue about cosmetic surgery, namely, that while a person is free to request such surgery, a doctor is not obliged to provide it, especially if the doctor feels that the risks of such surgery are too great. While one may make choices about the way one wishes to lead one's life, other people are not normally obligated to assist in the realization of those choices. However, if a person wishes to undergo a cosmetic surgical procedure, and if a suitably qualified doctor is willing to perform that procedure, then respect for autonomy would compel us to respect that choice.

A second way in which it might be argued that there is a difference between cosmetic surgery and other forms of bodily modification like tattooing would be to establish the rather tenuous premise that medicine is in some way fundamentally different from other forms of bodily modification, an argument well beyond the scope of this chapter. I will thus set this second argument aside and assume that if the exercise of autonomy can be used to justify practices such as tattooing and body piercing, then it can also be used to justify cosmetic surgery. The exception to this is if undergoing cosmetic surgery would cause harm to, or undermine the right to autonomy of, other moral agents. Thus as long as the provision or existence of cosmetic surgery does not cause harm or undermine the right to autonomy of people within society, then by virtue of their right to autonomy, people have a right to seek out and undergo cosmetic surgery procedures.

Therefore in order to provide an autonomy-based defense of cosmetic surgery, it is simply necessary to demonstrate that neither the existence of, nor the provision of, cosmetic surgery will cause harm to, or undermine the authority of, other moral agents. Since surgeons are not compelled to perform surgeries that they take to be unnecessarily risky, I cannot see how the provision of cosmetic surgery can undermine the autonomy of other moral agents, so it only remains to see if the provision of this type of surgery could be seen to cause harm to other agents.

The only obvious way in which it might be argued that the existence of, or provision of, cosmetic surgery might cause harm to other moral agents is to suggest that the provision of cosmetic surgery draws medical resources away from other, more important, forms of medicine. One way to answer this charge is to point out that an argument of this type can really only be applied to publicly funded medical services. Thus if cosmetic surgery is provided only as a private service, then such an argument does not apply. As a matter of fact, if one looks around the world, it can be seen that even private cosmetic surgery services are extremely unlikely to be offered unless other medical services are already seen to be adequately provided. It certainly appears that unless demand for other medical services is being adequately catered for, there is generally insufficient demand for cosmetic surgery for such services to be profitable.

In fact, denying people access to many forms of plastic surgery might actually be counterproductive in this regard, in that lack of access to certain forms of plastic surgery might actually lead to a greater drain on other medical services than if those plastic surgery services were available. Consider again, for example, the Dutch criteria for allowable publicly funded cosmetic surgery, specifically those cases where the patient is undergoing psychiatric treatment specifically for problems with appearance. Such psychiatric treatment is likely to be ongoing and will be reasonably expensive to provide in the longer term. Most important, such psychiatric treatment will be focused on the *symptoms* of the patient's problem, rather than on the *cause*. If this patient were able to have the cause of their problem treated, through plastic surgery, then this may well prove to be not only a more direct solution to the patient's problem but a more economical one as well.

There is one other extremely important way in which the autonomy-based defense of cosmetic surgery can be attacked, and that is through the suggestion that most (or perhaps all) of those people seeking cosmetic surgery are not in fact making an autonomous choice. If the people seeking cosmetic surgery have been coerced, duped, or manipulated or are in some other way unable to appropriately evaluate their values and commitments, then they cannot be said to be acting autonomously in choosing to seek cosmetic surgery. The practice of cosmetic surgery cannot be defended on the grounds of being necessary to uphold people's autonomy if no one is in fact autonomously choosing to undergo cosmetic surgery.

This is actually a common feminist response to cosmetic surgery. The argument suggests that women are duped by the false promises of the beauty myth and seek cosmetic surgery in an attempt to achieve the unattainable ideal of the perfect body. In other words, those who seek cosmetic surgery have been influenced by the culture in which they live—a culture with an emphasis on youth and beauty—in such a way that they are no longer able to adequately consider their own fundamental values and commitments. In the end, the values that they are acting upon in choosing to undergo cosmetic surgery are not their own values, but rather the values of the society in which they live.

I would suggest that there are serious problems with such an argument. By denying that the decision to choose cosmetic surgery is autonomous, those who advance this argument seem to me actually to be denying the moral agency of the people choosing cosmetic surgery, for if the cultural influences on these people are so strong that they make autonomous choices impossible with regard to the decision of whether or not to seek cosmetic surgery, then surely those same cultural influences will affect other decisions and make autonomous decisions impossible with regard to those decisions as well. How far do these influences extend, and how could one possibly prove that one was in fact making a well-considered decision that was not unduly influenced (except perhaps by making a decision that bucked the cultural trend)? In fact, it is difficult to suggest that these people are not acting autonomously in choosing cosmetic surgery without outright denial of autonomy—for isn't everyone going to be affected by the cultural concerns with which they live?

In order to consistently apply the argument that those who seek cosmetic surgery have been duped into making such a decision, it would appear necessary to raise those same questions about any person who made a decision to go along with any dominant cultural trend. Thus the only way to demonstrate autonomy, and to have one's choices accepted as being truly autonomous, would be to decide to act in a way that opposed those dominant cultural trends. While one might bemoan the existence of such strong cultural influences, particularly with regard to our current beauty culture, to use them as reason to deny the apparently autonomous choices of those choosing to go along with those dominant cultural trends seems to me to threaten to undermine the entire concept of autonomy.

## CONCLUSION

It has been my intention in this chapter to attempt to defend the practice of cosmetic surgery, through two main lines of argument. The first line of argument attempted to demonstrate that many forms of plastic surgery, rather than being undertaken for mere vanity reasons, are actually aimed at dealing with less obvious problems of the patient. This led me to question whether such surgeries really qualify as purely cosmetic surgery at all. My second line of argument was to mount a defense of the practice of cosmetic surgery through a focus on patient autonomy. I attempted to prove that the practice of cosmetic surgery does not divert needed resources away from other more fundamental forms of medical services, and I also argued that, while cultural influences on decisions to seek cosmetic surgery may be strong, suggesting that such influences prevent moral agents from making autonomous decisions risks undermining the entire concept of autonomy. Such strong cultural influences may well give us reason to attempt to modify the culture, but they do not give us reason to reject the autonomous decisions of those who choose to act in accordance with those influences.

## NOTES

My thanks to Nikki Coleman for her helpful comments on an earlier version of this chapter.

1. The following discussion of the funding of plastic surgery in the Netherlands draws heavily on Kathy Davis's *Dubious Equalities and Embodied Differences* (Lanham, MD: Rowman & Littlefield, 2003), 62–65.

2. Interestingly the "cost" of these procedures was discussed in exclusively monetary terms, with no mention of the time, pain, and risks that such surgery entailed.

3. Quoted in Karen S. Schneider, "Facing Off over Plastic Surgery," *Who* (Sydney), November 1, 2004, 38.

4. From *Die Aesthetische Chirurgie und ihre soziale Bedeutung*, quoted in Davis, *Dubious Equalities*, 27.

5. See Davis, *Dubious Equalities*, 44–45.

6. Davis devotes an entire chapter of her book to discussion of this issue. See *Dubious Equalities*, ch. 5, "Surgical Passing: Why Michael Jackson's Nose Makes 'Us' Uneasy."

7. See Davis, *Dubious Equalities*, 75–77.

8. My thanks to John Quilter for his insightful comments on this point.

9. I recognize that some people are likely to criticize such a definition of autonomy as being too thin, but I would defend myself on this point by noting that this is the way that autonomy is usually defined in bioethical discussions.

# 11

# Beauty under the Knife:
# A Feminist Appraisal of
# Cosmetic Surgery

## Rosemarie Tong and Hilde Lindemann

While roughly two-thirds of the plastic and reconstructive surgery done in the United States today is performed for therapeutic reasons, the other third is performed for aesthetic or cosmetic reasons to enhance one's appearance. As might be expected, however, the line between therapeutic and cosmetic surgery is blurred (Dibacco 1994). For burn victims, accident victims, or victims of violence, for example, the goal is not only to replace damaged tissue and to repair damaged body parts but also to give the patient an acceptable appearance. Nevertheless, there is a difference between undergoing rhinoplasty to relieve one's breathing problems and having the surgery to improve one's already acceptable appearance.

Cosmetic surgery is, like most surgery, somewhat risky. In fact, the American Society of Plastic and Reconstructive Surgeons (ASPRS) publishes a pamphlet on cosmetic surgery, the contents of which could easily raise doubts in potential patients' minds about the wisdom of elective procedures. Not only does this ASPRS pamphlet discuss possibilities such as infection, bleeding, blood clots, scarring, and adverse reactions to anesthesia but it also notes, for example, that liposuction can trigger a shock-inducing excessive loss of fluid and that face-lifts can cause injury to the nerves that control facial muscles. The same pamphlet indicates that breast augmentation surgery is also not without risk: it can result in conditions ranging from tightening and hardening of scar tissue around the implant to the rupturing of the implant (ASPRS 1993, 3).

In addition to entailing some risks, most cosmetic procedures are relatively expensive and not covered by health insurance unless they are performed for a therapeutic purpose. Liposuction, for instance, costs anywhere from $2,600 to $10,000, and its cousin, the tummy tuck, costs around $8,000.

For breast augmentation, surgical fees alone (not counting anesthesia, operating room facilities, and other related expenses) run between $3,000 and $7,000. Compared to some cosmetic procedures, however, such one-time expenses might seem like a bargain. Many women are advised to get their first face-lift at the age of 40 and to pay anywhere from $5,500 to $14,500 every 5 to 15 years thereafter to have surgery repeated. Similarly, collagen injections usually last only a few months to one year and cost around $375 each time.[1]

Given its risks and costs, many people simply assume that only the rich and famous go in for cosmetic surgery. This commonsense assumption proves to be a false one, however. Almost 70 percent of the people who elect to have cosmetic surgery have family incomes of less than $40,000 per year.[2] Ordinary people—hairdressers, grocery store clerks, and secretaries—as well as movie stars, millionaires, and models are willing to spend a considerable portion of their incomes redesigning their bodies, particularly their faces.

## TRADITIONAL FEMINIST CRITICISMS OF COSMETIC SURGERY

From roughly 1975 to 1995, many feminists opposed cosmetic surgery on the grounds that the practice reinforced the oppressive power relation that goes by the name of gender. For the most part, these feminists did not object to therapeutic plastic and reconstructive surgery aimed at removing or repairing the kind of birth defects and developmental abnormalities that cause people to avert their eyes from someone. Nor was their quarrel with surgery whose purpose was to remove or repair acquired deformities, including those resulting from trauma (domestic violence) or disease (breast cancer). Rather, their objection was to the use of plastic and reconstructive surgery for nonmedical purposes, specifically for the purpose of making women look younger and more beautiful.

The fact that many men also underwent cosmetic surgery for nonmedical purposes did not convince the feminists described above that the practice was gender neutral (Devine 1995). Although some men were pressured to get chin, eye, and/or nose jobs in order to look leaner and meaner at the workplace, most men found that they could get by in life—indeed, do very well—without ever visiting a cosmetic surgeon's office. However, the same could not be said for most women, in Kathryn Pauly Morgan's estimation. She claimed that with few exceptions, cosmetic surgery is required for women in ways that it is not required for men.

As cosmetic surgery becomes increasingly normalized through the concept of female "make-over" that is translated into columns and articles in the print media or made into nationwide television shows directed at female viewers, as the "success stories" are invited on the talk shows along with their "makers," and as surgically transformed women enter the Miss America pageants, women who refuse to submit to the knives and to the needles, to the anesthetics and the bandages, will come to be seen as deviant in one way or another. Women who refuse to use these technologies are already becoming stigmatized as "unliberated," not caring about their appearance (a sign of disturbed gender identity and low self-esteem according to various health-care professionals), as "refusing to be all that they could be" or as "granola-heads." (Morgan 1991, 40)

Sandra Lee Bartky added to Morgan's observations some insightful remarks about how U.S. society in particular uses women's body image to control women's behavior. She wrote:

Women are no longer required to be chaste or modest, to restrict their sphere of activity to the home, or even to realize their properly feminine destiny in maternity. Normative femininity [that is, the rules for being a good woman] is coming more and more to be centered on woman's body—not its duties and obligations or even its capacity to bear children, but its sexuality, more precisely, its presumed heterosexuality and its appearance. . . . The woman who checks her makeup half a dozen times a day to see if her foundation has caked or her mascara has run, who worries that the wind or the rain may spoil her hairdo, who looks frequently to see if her stockings have bagged at the ankle, or who, feeling fat, monitors everything she eats, has become, just as surely as the inmate of Panopticon, a self-policing subject, a self committed to a relentless self-surveillance. This self-surveillance is a form of obedience to patriarchy. (Bartky 1990, 81)

An additional issue that troubled feminists throughout the 1970s, 1980s, and early 1990s was that of who performs most of the cosmetic surgeries in the United States. Although more women are choosing dermatology or plastic and reconstructive surgery as their specialty in medical school, their numbers are relatively small in comparison to the men who make the same choice. The preponderance of U.S. board-certified plastic and reconstructive surgeons are men, and despite the fact that men have cosmetic surgery too, most of those who elect it are female. This situation reaffirms an existing hierarchy of women going to men in positions of authority for appraisal and correction of their "flawed" bodies. It also reaffirms a social given, in that women's choices are seen to be more legitimate when supported by or carried out in concert with men, as the male perspective is seen as more rational and authoritative.

Over and beyond Morgan's "Women and the Knife" and Bartky's "Foucault, Femininity, and the Modernization of Patriarchal Power," other well-known examples of feminist disapproval of cosmetic surgery throughout the last few decades include Naomi Wolf's *The Beauty Myth*, Susan Bordo's *Unbearable Weight*, and Elizabeth Haiken's *Venus Envy*. Their position regarding cosmetic surgery, and more generally the female body and its place in society, was that the tyranny of slenderness and youthful appearance symbolized by this surgery is a negative and harmful aspect of American and Western culture.

For Wolf, cosmetic surgery is an example of the "institutionalized forms of power working in concert to force women into extreme beauty practices."[3] As she saw it, women's need throughout the world, (and particularly in developed Western nations) to be beautiful, and the forms that this need takes, is "the result of nothing more exalted than the need in today's power structure, economy, and culture to mount a counteroffensive against women" (Wolf 1991, 13). In addition, women's beauty serves as the foundation of women's identity and leaves them "vulnerable to outside approval" and vulnerable to the need for increasingly invasive ways to stay beautiful (14). Specifically regarding cosmetic surgery, Wolf stated that it is a market that has been created not because of an actual need for the surgery, but for surgeons to make money and as a way of keeping women politically and socially immobilized as they squander time worrying about their perceived "flaws"—time that could be spent on pursuing and achieving educational and occupational goals. As she put it, "Modern cosmetic surgeons have a direct financial interest in a social role for women that requires them to feel ugly" (223).

Noting that women's success depends on their good looks to a far greater degree than men's success does, many feminists in the 1970s, 1980s, and 1990s acknowledged that it was not illogical for the average woman to reason that if "dressing for success" made sense, then so did cosmetic surgery for success. In the estimation of Bordo (1993, 20), women who reasoned in this way were "neither dupes nor critics of sexist culture" but simply individuals who wanted to do well in it. They elected cosmetic surgery not because they were "passively taken in by media norms" but precisely because they had "correctly discerned that these norms shape the perceptions and desires of potential lovers and employers." Far from being embarrassed by their decision to undergo cosmetic surgery, Bordo noted, many of these women regarded themselves as feminists. They viewed themselves as strong women who could "play the game" exceedingly well and use their bodies to achieve their goals.

To be sure, feminists like Morgan, Bartky, Wolf, and Bordo very much doubted that women who deliberately behave in ways that bolster patriarchy can, in good conscience, call themselves feminists. As they saw it, *true* feminists are committed to *resisting* the imperatives of sexist culture. Specifically, they are committed to helping women see the extent to which women are controlled by socially constructed ideals about female beauty—ideals that, because they are overall unattainable, make women feel perpetually badly about themselves, no matter how successful they are in the domestic realm or in the workplace. Bartky provided the telling example of the successful singer Dinah Shore to bolster the claim that no woman is impervious to the force of the Beauty Myth. She quoted Shore:

One of the many things men don't understand about women is the extent to which our self-esteem depends on how we feel we look at any given moment—and how much we yearn for a compliment, at any age. If I had just won the Nobel Peace Prize but felt my hair looked awful, I would not be glowing with self-assurance when I entered the room. (Bartky 1990, 33)

## EMERGING REASSESSMENTS OF COSMETIC SURGERY: WHAT DO WOMEN THEMSELVES SAY?

Among the issues about resistance that feminist critics of cosmetic surgery in the 1970s, 1980s, and 1990s never resolved was *how much* resistance to the forces of beauty was required for "true" feminists. Was it enough to resist seriously risky, invasive, and extensive cosmetic surgery elected solely for the purpose of remaining attractive in the eyes of men? Or did one also have to resist relatively risk-free and minor cosmetic surgeries (for example, aggressive skin treatments) elected mainly for the purpose of having clean and healthy-looking skin? Indeed, was one required to resist any and all beautifying or anti-aging products and procedures for fear of reinforcing the view that unless a woman was young and beautiful she was of little value?

Taken to its extreme—that is, to the point of deliberately making one's self ugly to defy the Beauty Myth—most women, including most feminists, came to the conclusion that true feminism was accommodating enough to embrace women who liked "looking good," dressing up, wearing makeup, and even getting a "nip and tuck" here and there. Beginning in the early 1990s, feminists became less interested in telling women what they had to do in order to be free and happy and more interested in simply listening to what women themselves say about their struggles to be free and happy. As Suzanne Fraser put it, it is necessary to examine "the range of ways in which women speak of their motives and their feelings about themselves. . . . Generalizations about motives are untenable" (2003, 3). She, Debra Gimlin, and Kathy Davis have all conducted empirical studies of how women who have undergone cosmetic surgery speak about it, both before and after the procedure.

In listening to women who choose cosmetic surgery, Gimlin found a sharp contrast between what they saw themselves as doing and what theorists took them to be doing. In her 2002 article "Cosmetic Surgery: Paying for Your Beauty," Gimlin wrote:

Cosmetic surgery stands, for many theorists and social critics, as the ultimate invasion of the human body for the sake of physical beauty. It epitomizes the astounding lengths to which contemporary women will go to obtain bodies that meet current ideals of attractiveness. As such, plastic surgery is perceived by many to be qualitatively different from aerobics, hair styling, or even dieting. In

this view, cosmetic surgery is not about controlling one's own body but is instead an activity so extreme, so invasive that it can only be interpreted as subjugation. (95)

In this view, the women who undergo cosmetic surgery are reproducing
"some of the worst aspects of the beauty culture, not so much through the
act of the surgery itself as through their ideological efforts to restore appearance as an indicator of character." After having listened to what women
themselves say about why they opted for surgery, however, Gimlin rejects
the social critics' position. "I am not convinced," she writes, "that reducing
facial wrinkles is somehow less 'real' than dyeing hair from gray to brown
or even that eye surgery or rhinoplasty is somehow less authentic than a decision to have straight rather than curly hair" (107).

Gimlin found that many women who elected cosmetic surgery were quite
able to control their need for it. The women she interviewed were not ad-
dicted to cosmetic surgery. None of them were like the often-interviewed
women who have had one surgery after another so that they could achieve
their goal of looking exactly like the doll Barbie: wasp-waisted, full-breasted,
and blonde. And none of them thought that cosmetic surgery could or
should entirely transform their appearance. On the contrary, the women
with whom Gimlin spoke seemed content to use cosmetic surgery to address
a particular "flaw" rather than to attain some sort of ideal beauty. They
stressed that they did not get surgery to please others but to please themselves or to approximate more closely their own vision of themselves (96,
106–7).

Significantly, in a book just as full of interviews as Gimlin's, Kathy Davis
concurs with Gimlin's observations repeatedly. As she puts it in her 1995 *Reshaping the Female Body: The Dilemma of Cosmetic Surgery* (3–5), "Cosmetic surgery was clearly more complicated than I had imagined. I had previously associated it either with well-to-do American housewives who were bored
with their suburban lives and wanted to have a face-lift or with the celebrity
'surgical junkies' who couldn't seem to stop remaking their bodies," not
feminist friends who understood the dangers and the cultural implications
of cosmetic surgery. Davis reveals to her readers how she was initially
thrown when her friend, who, as she puts it, is "critical of the suffering
women have to endure because their bodies do not meet the normative requirements of feminine beauty," nevertheless decided to have cosmetic surgery *"for herself"* (emphasis in original). She confesses that, for a while, she
doubted whether her friend was a feminist at all; but she gradually concluded that for her friend, cosmetic surgery made good sense. Her friend
was having the surgery to please herself and cosmetic surgery was giving
her the opportunity "to renegotiate her relationship to her body and through
her body to the world around her." Davis's friend experienced herself not as
"just a body" that had to conform to others' expectations, but as "a subject

with a body" that she could use to express herself to others. If one can change one's ways of thinking, why cannot one change one's way of looking?

Gimlin and Davis concede that in obtaining a face-lift, a woman might not be delighting herself but simply doing the best she can in an environment that is sexist, ageist, and deeply moralistic about physical appearance. One of the women Gimlin interviews supports this point when she discusses getting cosmetic surgery to deal with "pressures in 'the workfield.'" As this woman explained, "Despite the fact that we have laws against age discrimination, employers do find ways of getting around it. I know women my age who do not get jobs or are relieved of jobs because of age" (2002, 100). Davis likewise emphasizes that many of the women who get cosmetic surgery are, perhaps, "exercising power under conditions which are not of one's own making. In the context of limited possibilities for action, cosmetic surgery can be a way for an individual woman to give shape to her life by reshaping her body. . . . For a woman whose suffering has gone beyond a certain point, cosmetic surgery can become a matter of justice—the only fair thing to do" (1995, 163).

Davis usefully suggests that cosmetic surgery might be seen as "a dilemma rather than a form of self-inflicted subordination" and that in this way we can "understand what makes it both desirable *and* problematic for so many women" (180, emphasis in original). To see it this way is to recognize that here, as in so many other aspects of their lives, women are faced with a double bind. To ignore the norms that gender imposes on women's appearance is costly: it can play a role in the loss of a promotion, how seriously one is taken in the workplace or elsewhere, and the level of one's income. On the other hand, to conform to the norms of gender helps to perpetuate them, which can also play a role in the loss of a promotion, how seriously one is taken in the workplace or elsewhere, and the level of one's income. Given the damned-if-I-do, damned-if-I-don't nature of the decision to undergo cosmetic surgery and the complicated feelings and beliefs many women have about their bodies, Davis concludes that "a concern for the complexity of women's desire to have cosmetic surgery makes it difficult to come up with either a blanket rejection or a gratifying resolution to the problems of cosmetic surgery" (181).

## EMERGING FEMINIST THEORIES ON COSMETIC SURGERY: HONORING WHAT WOMEN WANT

"The emphasis on feminine beauty," Ann J. Cahill observes in a recent article, "is a controlling force in women's lives, and the fact that some individual women claim to be choosing aspects of beautification independently does not necessarily contradict its role in perpetuating sexual inequality. In a word, then, pleasure in feminine beautification can neither be dismissed outright nor uncritically endorsed" (2003, 43). Instead, Cahill urges us to acknowledge that practices aimed at enhancing women's appearance involve "negotiation among a variety of discourses and imperatives" (51).

Cahill argues that for different women there are different limits to beautification, and the question is whether "participation in socially demanded forms of beautification necessarily" hinders "women's ability to function as equal, autonomous beings" (42). At different points in time and in different settings, a woman who beautifies herself in a variety of ways can both experience "a social lessening of her agency" and find that involving herself in certain beautification processes (going to a hair or nail salon) has strengthened the bonds between herself and other women (60).

There is a subversive element to female beautification, in that some women can use the time that they work to beautify themselves or have others beautify them as a time to bond with other women and to improve and build upon female relationships. Indeed, in her study of older women's conversations in beauty parlors, Frida Furman (1997) finds that important ties of friendship and community are forged during these rituals of beautification. Cahill notes that there are "pleasures" when "feminine beautification" is "more than an attempt to overcome or answer the lack associated with the feminine body by a patriarchal society" (2003, 46). She speaks of "specific ways in which beautification practices can create a communal experience that furthers feminist aims," noting that "the time devoted to the process of beautification indicates not its oppressive nature but its potential for feminist agency" (43, 52).

For Cahill, beautification generally and cosmetic surgery specifically become problematic only when they stop being useful to a woman's independence, freedom, and autonomy. As with many feminists of the new millennium, Cahill seems more comfortable with women beautifying themselves to suit social norms and cultural expectations as well as themselves than were feminists writing in the 1970s, 1980s, and 1990s. The fact that a woman uses makeup, has cosmetic surgery, wears sexually provocative clothes, or sells her sexual services is no longer taken as a sure sign that she has demeaned, diminished, or otherwise objectified herself. It has come to seem possible that, on the contrary, such a woman pairs the "trappings of traditional femininity or sexuality" with "demonstrations of strength or power" (Bailey 2002, 145).

The danger, of course, is that contemporary understandings of these matters could fail to take seriously the idea that gender *requires* women to be preoccupied with their looks and femininity. Amy Richards, coauthor of *Manifesta: Young Women, Feminism, and the Future*, stated in an interview: "I don't think these women are saying 'I'm going to be female, going be objectified, going to wear sexy clothes and so on and be part of the backlash against feminism.' I think they're saying, 'I'm going to do all these things because I want to embrace my femininity'" (Bailey 2002, 144). It is easy, when participating in practices of beautification, to lose sight of the fact that femininity is a social construction working to the systemic advantage of men and the systemic disadvantage of women. To "sound female" and carry oneself in feminine ways requires constant, habitual self-monitoring. There are daily, costly, time-consuming activities involved in being a woman: a feminine body "must constantly reassure its audience by a willing demonstration of difference, even when one does not exist in nature" (Brownmiller 1984, 15).

The dangers notwithstanding, Ann Braithwaite reminds us that 2005 is a very different time from 1975. As she puts it:

> An engagement with . . . practices of seemingly traditional femininity does not necessarily carry the same meanings for young women today or for the culture they live in that they might have to earlier feminist periods, and thus cannot be the point upon which to write off specific cultural practices as somehow apolitical and therefore "post-" or "anti-" feminist. (2002, 340)

For Cathryn Bailey, the fact that younger feminists are focusing on their femininity is "a wake-up call for older feminists that what appears, from one perspective, to be conformist, may, from another perspective, have subversive potential. . . . We cannot assess the meaning of younger women's actions and attitudes without recognizing that the backdrop against which their actions are performed is, in many cases, significantly different" (2002, 145).

Marcelle Karp and Debbie Stoller likewise argue that "the trappings of femininity could be used to make a sexual statement that was powerful, rather than passive" (1999, 45):

> Unlike our feminist foremothers, who claimed that makeup was the opiate of the misses, we're positively prochoice when it comes to matters of feminine display. We're well aware . . . of the beauty myth that's working to keep women obscene and not heard, but we just don't think that transvestites should have all the fun. . . . We love our lipstick, have a passion for polish, and, adore this armor that we call "fashion." To us, it's fun, it's feminine, and, in the particular way we flaunt it, it's definitely feminist. (47)

Jennifer Baumgardner and Amy Richards echo these sentiments in *Manifesta*. As they explain, "The cultural and social weapons that had been identified (rightly so) in the Second Wave as instruments of oppression—women as sex objects, fascist fashion, pornographic materials—are no longer being exclusively wielded against women and are sometimes wielded by women" (2000, 141). They believe that women in general are much more conscious of the ways in which their bodies are used against them and that they often put these bodies and the stereotypes to their own uses, to gain their own power.

Even if gender requires women to look young and beautiful to a far greater degree than it requires men to look good, and even if it punishes women for "letting themselves go," some women nonetheless might choose cosmetic surgery not because they or others feel they are worth nothing without it, nor because they fear that they might lose their husbands or jobs, but simply because they would like to look better than they do. Others, rightly supposing that it is easier to change one's physical appearance than to shift entrenched social attitudes and topple unjust power systems, might prefer the surgery to nastier forms of discrimination. In our deeply gendered society, a woman cannot know whether her decision to undergo cosmetic surgery will really further her own or other women's interests in freedom and well-being (Bartky 1990, 62). All that she can do is ponder the matter from a feminist political and ethical point of view and hope that, on balance, her decision to use cosmetic surgery will not frustrate her own or other women's ability to live well and fully.

## NOTES

1. See, for example, prices advertised at the San Francisco Plastic Surgery and Laser Center, http://www.sfcosmeticsurgery.com/costs/index.htm, or the Liposuction Cosmetic Surgery Center, http://www.liposuction-cosmetic-surgery.com/costs.htm. Statistics for 2003 (the most recent year for which they are available) are kept by the American Society of Plastic and Reconstructive Surgeons and can be viewed at http://www.plasticsurgery.org/public_education/2003statistics.cfm.
2. American Society of Plastic and Reconstructive Surgeons, statistics for 2003.
3. Wolf, quoted in Fraser 2003, 100.

## REFERENCES

ASPRS [American Society of Plastic and Reconstructive Surgeons]. 1993. *Plastic surgery and to-tal patient care.* Arlington Heights, IL: ASPRS.
Bailey, Cathryn. 2002. Unpacking the mother/daughter baggage: Reassessing second- and third-wave tensions. *Women's Studies Quarterly* 30 (3–4): 138–54.
Bartky, Sandra Lee. 1990. *Femininity and domination: Studies in the phenomenology of oppression.* New York: Routledge.
Baumgardner, Jennifer, and Amy Richards. 2000. *Manifesta: Young women, feminism, and the future.* New York: Farrar, Straus and Giroux.
Bordo, Susan. 1993. *Unbearable weight: Feminism, Western culture, and the body.* Berkeley: University of California Press.
Braithwaite, Ann. 2002. The personal, the political, third-wave and postfeminisms. *Feminist Theory* 3 (3): 340.
Brownmiller, Susan, 1984. *Femininity.* New York: Fawcett Columbine.
Cahill, Ann J. 2003. Feminist pleasure and feminine beautification. *Hypatia* 18 (4): 42–64.
Davis, Kathy. 1995. *Reshaping the female body: The dilemma of cosmetic surgery.* New York: Routledge.
Devine, M. 1995. Looking your best. *St. Paul Magazine,* February, 164.
Dibacco, T. V. 1994. Altered images. *Washington Post.* 13 December, Health section.
Fraser, Suzanne. 2003. *Cosmetic surgery, gender and culture.* New York: Palgrave MacMillan.

Furman, Frida K. 1997. *Facing the mirror: Older women and beauty shop culture.* New York: Routledge.

Gimlin, Debra L., ed. 2002. *Body work: Beauty and self-image in American culture.* Berkeley: University of California Press.

Haiken, Elizabeth. 1997. *Venus envy: A history of cosmetic surgery.* Baltimore: Johns Hopkins University Press.

Karp, Marcelle, and Debbie Stoller. 1999. *The bust guide to the new girl order.* New York : Penguin Books.

Morgan, Kathryn Pauly. 1991. Women and the knife: Cosmetic surgery and the colonization of women's bodies. *Hypatia* 6 (3): 25–53.

Wolf, Naomi. 1991. *The beauty myth: How images of beauty are used against women.* New York: William Morrow.

# VI

# PLACEBO SURGERY

The Emperor's New Scar: The Ethics of Placebo Surgery
*David Neil*

Sham Surgery and Reasonable Risks
*Alex John London*

# 12

# The Emperor's New Scar:
# The Ethics of Placebo Surgery

*David Neil*

Surgical innovation is something of a gray area in medical research. Relative to other doctors, surgeons exercise a high degree of discretion in the trialing of new techniques with their patients. The first patients to undergo a new procedure are, in a real sense, subjects in an experiment. It is always hoped that a new procedure will deliver a clinical benefit, but as often as not, trial means error. The frontline patients bear a higher burden of risk, with lower expectation of success than subsequent patients, who benefit from the experience gained in the early attempts.

While experimentation is as intrinsic to the progress of surgery as any other field of medicine, nowhere is surgical innovation regulated by the kinds of guidelines and oversight required in other human experimentation. In one recent study, Angelique Reitsma and Jonathan Moreno identified 59 papers in U.S. medical journals between 1992 and 2000 that described innovative surgery. They then sent a questionnaire to the papers' authors. Of those surgeons who responded, the majority had not submitted their proposal to an institutional review board (IRB) and a majority had not mentioned the innovative nature of the procedure on the informed consent form. Two-thirds of the respondents stated that government regulation for the protection of human subjects of innovative surgical research would not be appropriate. Reitsma and Moreno locate the source of these surgeons' attitudes in a tradition in surgery whereby new techniques, and even new devices, "are regarded as mere modifications and not as research" (2002, 793). Thus surgical innovations often bypass processes in place to protect human subjects. Elsewhere, the same authors have noted:

> The majority of surgical publications involve interventional case reports that consist of a series of patients; outcome measures are usually clinical parameters

that are obtained during routine clinical follow-up, without any type of formal written protocol. The implicit assumption in these case reports is that the clinical hypothesis is not formalized until *after* the therapeutic intervention. These types of "informal research" are viewed as clinical care and are therefore invisible to IRBs. (Reitsma and Moreno 2003, 49–50)

This kind of informal surgical research is at odds with the increasing trend toward evidence-based medicine. Concerns about the evidential basis for procedures is not limited to novel techniques. Many procedures that were once common have since been abandoned when more rigorous evaluation has disproved their presumed benefits—routine tonsillectomy, to name one (Freeman et al. 1999). Suppose we accept that, in principle, there is a clear need for more rigorous and objective standards for assessing new surgical procedures. In practice, this will mean randomized control trials—and this is ethically problematic because, unlike placebo sugar pills, surgical placebos are not benign.

Randomized, double-blind, placebo-controlled trials are widely recognized as the gold standard for drug trials. Such trials are the most effective way to control for both investigator bias and the placebo effect. A few surgical trials have also been conducted with a placebo control. Patients on the placebo arm of the trial receive "sham" or "imitation" surgery (as it is sometimes called) such that the patient cannot know whether she received the trial procedure or not. Placebo surgery typically involves anesthesia and an incision equivalent to the incision needed for the actual surgery. To maximize equivalence between the trial and control groups, it may also involve the same postoperative drug therapy given to the recipients of the "real" surgery. These trials have proven highly controversial. Placebo surgery obviously involves risks that are not there with placebo pills.

Critics of placebo-controlled surgical trials (PCST) claim that such trials are straightforwardly unethical because they violate the doctor's duty to act only in the best interests of the patient (Clark 2002). These trials expose patients to some of the normal risks of surgery without any reasonable expectation of benefit.

Defenders of PCST point to their considerable scientific value. They argue that without properly designed trials for new procedures, we cannot identify false positives and determine their real effectiveness, and in some cases well-designed clinical trials require a placebo control (Albin 2002).

The use of placebo surgery to control for the placebo effect in the evaluation of surgical procedures was first advocated by Henry Beecher (1961). Beecher discussed two PCST, conducted in the late 1950s, to test the efficacy of ligation of the internal mammary artery for the treatment of angina, a common treatment at the time. Both trials showed that the procedure was no more effective than the placebo, and the operation was subsequently abandoned. These two trials together enrolled 35 subjects and probably prevented thousands of unnecessary operations (Albin 2002, 323).

We will examine here two more-recent trials that have generated some controversy, beginning with a brief description of these trials.

## FETAL CELL TRANSPLANTS FOR PARKINSON'S DISEASE

Parkinson's disease is a motor function disorder characterized by tremors, rigidity, slowness of movement, impaired gait, and loss of balance and postural stability. Its main pathological feature is a loss of dopamine-producing neurons in a particular area of the brain. The drug Levadopa (a dopamine precursor) is the standard treatment. It is effective at controlling symptoms in the early and middle stages of the disease, but is often ineffective in advanced patients, and the higher doses needed have serious side effects. In animal models, it has been shown that "dopaminergic neurons" harvested from embryos and transplanted to the damaged areas can to some extent regrow the damaged neural structures and reverse the loss of motor control. The transplantation of embryonic cells into the brains of human sufferers has been undertaken in a number of centers around the world; one study reports around 360 transplant procedures at 17 centers as of 1999 (Clark 2002, 60). Results have been mixed, but some centers have claimed to consistently produce significant improvement in patients.

However, strong and persistent placebo effects have been reported in the treatment of Parkinson's disease. In one large, double-blind drug trial, patients in the placebo group had a 20–30 percent improvement in motor scores, persisting throughout the six months of the trial (Freeman et al. 1999). Because of the wide variations in response to drugs for Parkinson's disease, placebo effects are a major issue in the evaluation of new drugs. Consequently it is possible that the claimed clinical benefits of fetal tissue transplants for Parkinson's disease are also a placebo effect, or are exaggerated by investigator bias.

One reason the procedure has always been highly controversial is that the fetal tissue is obtained from aborted fetuses 6.5 to 9 weeks old, but concerns relating to the moral status of embryos are not at issue here. In the United States, a ban on federal support for the medical use of fetal tissue was lifted by President Clinton in 1993. The National Institutes of Health subsequently agreed to fund two randomized control trials to assess the efficacy of the procedure.

The first trial involved 40 patients with advanced Parkinson's disease, for whom drug therapy had become ineffective (Freed et al. 2001). The patients were randomly allocated to receive either the transplant or a placebo operation. Each transplant patient received tissue taken from four fetuses, injected into the damaged areas on both sides of the brain. For the patients given the placebo procedure—that is, not receiving the fetal tissue—the risks and discomforts included a local anesthetic, the placing of stereotactic equipment, a scalp incision, and the drilling of burr holes (not all the way through the skull). This study reported no significant difference between the transplant and the placebo groups. (Unfortunately, in five of the transplant patients, the grafts grew *too* well and these patients suffered uncontrollable involuntary movements and muscle spasms, probably due to an excess of dopamine.)

The second Parkinson's trial was designed to address some questions raised by the first one, concerning immunological effects and the comparison of different amounts of transplant tissue (Fletcher 2003). This trial had three arms. In the first, patients received tissue from four fetal sources. Patients in the second arm received a smaller amount of tissue from just one fetus. The third arm was the placebo control group. The patients on the placebo arm faced the risks of a general anesthetic, low-dose immunosuppresant therapy (cyclosporine), and the radioisotopes used in brain imaging, as well as all the other risks present in the earlier trial.

The published results of this second trial showed no overall treament effect. There was early improvement in some of the patients with less severe symptoms who received the higher amount of fetal tissue. However, 13 of the transplant patients (more than half) developed *dyskenesias* (uncontrollable movement), and three of them needed further surgery to relieve this serious side effect. Subjects enrolled in the trial were told that if they received the placebo, and the transplants subsequently proved safe and effective, they would then be offered the procedure at no cost. In a paper published in advance of the trial, aiming to justify the trial design, the experimenters listed the risks described above, the measures taken to minimize those risks, and described the benefits thus:

> The benefits of participating in the placebo group include contributing to advances in the treatment of a disease of great personal interest to the participants, receiving standard medical treatment at no cost, having the opportunity to obtain a fetal-tissue transplant at no cost if the procedure proves to be safe and effective, and being spared the risks associated with transplantation if it proves to be unsafe or ineffective. (Freeman et al. 1999)

In fact, the trials showed a higher than expected mortality rate, a high rate of serious side effects, and a significant placebo effect such that there was no statistically significant difference in benefits for the transplant group and the trial group. The results give rise to serious doubts about a procedure that has been undergone by hundreds of patients.

## ARTHROSCOPIC SURGERY
## FOR OSTEOARTHRITIS OF THE KNEE

Patients with osteoarthritis of the knee, and for whom medical therapy has failed to relieve the pain, often choose to undergo one of two surgical procedures: arthroscopic lavage or débridement. The lavage procedure involves flushing the joint with at least 10 liters of fluid through arthroscopic cannulas, in order to remove debris. The débridement procedure is usually performed after lavaging the joint and involves shaving away rough cartilage and trimming torn or degenerated meniscal fragments, then smoothing the remaining meniscus. A study conducted in Texas assessed both surgical procedures against a placebo (Moseley et al. 2002).

In this study, a total of 180 patients were randomly assigned to arthroscopic débridement, arthroscopic lavage, or placebo surgery. All the procedures were performed by one surgeon. Patients were assessed over a 24-month period after surgery to assess improvements in pain and function. The surgeons had no role in the follow-up assessment of the patients, and the assessors were blinded to the treatment group assignment. For the placebo surgery, patients did not receive a standard general anesthetic, but instead were given an intravenous tranquilizer and an opioid, which is safer. Three one-centimeter incisions were made, and a débridement procedure was simulated, but no arthroscopic instruments were inserted into the knee. All patients spent the night after the procedure in the hospital, and their nurses were unaware of the treatment group assignment. There were two minor postoperative complications in the placebo group: one patient developed a wound infection, which was treated with antibiotics, and another developed calf swelling in the leg that had undergone surgery. Patients in all three groups received the same follow-up care: the same walking aids, the same exercise program, and the same analgesics.

The study found that the outcomes for both surgical procedures were no better than those after a placebo procedure. The authors concluded that, if their findings are correct, "the billions of dollars spent on such procedures annually might be put to better use" (Moseley et al. 2002, 87).[1]

## THE DILEMMA OF PLACEBO SURGERY

The moral dilemma presented by PCST is an instructive instance of the kind of dilemma that arises when the imperatives of research are in tension with the imperatives of clinical care. The real source of this dilemma is that the competing normative considerations are grounded in distinct and opposed ethical theories. The claim that doctors have an inviolable obligation to act only in the best interests of their patients appeals to a deontic conception of patients' rights and doctors' duties. However the doctor's duty to do what is "best" for her patient has an implicit temporal index. The object of the duty is a particular, present patient and the duty of care is a duty to offer that patient treatment in accordance with *current* medical wisdom about best practice. The object of research, however, is not any particular patient but a condition in general. Research on therapies assumes that current best practice is not necessarily the best possible practice and aims to provide future patients with more effective therapies than are presently available.

For the most part, we cannot say which individuals will benefit from to-day's research. Research brings benefits to a class of people—future Parkinson's patients, for instance—and for this reason, the justification of research typically appeals to utilitarian arguments. From a utilitarian perspective, dangers to research subjects can be justified when the potential benefits of new medical knowledge sufficiently outweigh the unavoidable risks of the research needed to gain that knowledge. In the case of surgical research, however, the surgeon is both researcher and treating doctor, and the moral requirements of both roles are not easily reconciled.

In an influential article, Ruth Macklin (1999) characterizes the dilemma as one "between the highest standard of research design and the highest standard of ethics." It is misleading, I think, to describe the problem as a tension between good science and good ethics, as if the only ethical considerations concern the protection of research subjects. If the benefits of good science did not carry moral weight—if *all* the ethical reasons pulled in one direction—then there would be no moral dilemma. Certainly, historically, the principal concern of research ethics has been the protection of subjects. However, the time frame over which research results are ultimately incorporated into standard practice is such that much medical research does not *directly* benefit the experimental subjects; so, if research ethics is *only* about the protection of subjects, then most medical research would be unjustifiable. The most effective way to minimize harms caused by research would simply be to do no research. In reality, the approval process for research proposals standardly involves judgments about the importance of the research in terms of future benefits. For the most part, what justifies risks imposed on research subjects is the utility of the knowledge to be gained, and much of the ambiguity in research ethics arises from the fact that there are no widely accepted methods for ethically evaluating these trade-offs.

Macklin compares PCST to placebo-controlled drug trials and finds that the justification for the latter cannot be extended to the former. Experimental drugs are normally trialed against the current standard treatment. It is considered acceptable to use a placebo control only when a drug is being trialed for a condition for which there is no effective drug available.

> The chief reason [why PCST is unethical] is that performing a surgical procedure that has no expected benefit other than the placebo effect violates the ethical and regulatory principle that the risk of harm to subjects must be minimized in the conduct of research. . . . It is undeniable that performing surgery in research subjects that has no potential therapeutic benefit fails to minimize the risk of harm. An alternative research design that did not involve sham surgery would pose a lower risk of harm to the subjects in the control group of the study. But herein lies the tension between the scientific and ethical standards: the alternative design would be less rigorous from a methodologic point of view. (Macklin 1999)

This argument is too quick and the problem lies in the ambiguity of the meaning of "minimizing risk." If "minimizing risk *to research subjects*" is construed in an unrestricted sense, then risks are minimized by doing no research. Of course, that is not the sense in play here. The relevant notion of "minimizing risk" is relational and has determinate content only relative to a specified objective. The power of a study determines the confidence with which general conclusions may be inferred from the experimental results. Uncontroversially, for any given study, we want the safest possible study design. If two candidate study designs will answer the same question with the same confidence level, the design carrying the least risk is to be rationally preferred. Two studies that cannot answer the same question with the same confidence are effectively two different studies. One study may involve less risk than another in an absolute sense, but "minimizing" does not just mean "lessening." One does not minimize the risks of football by deciding to play checkers instead. It is important not to confuse the idea of "minimizing risk," in the sense of finding the safest design for a study, with the distinct question of whether the best achievable risk–benefit balance for a proposed study is ultimately acceptable or unacceptable.

Macklin's argument has been criticized by Franklin Miller (2003), in an article defending the claim that PCST (or "sham surgery," as he calls it) can sometimes be justified. Miller rejects Macklin's understanding of the requirement to minimize risk, along similar lines to the criticism above. But Miller's defense of PCST is flawed. His main charge is that critics of PCST are "conflating the ethics of clinical research with the ethics of clinical care." Miller accepts the argument that, "judged by the surgical standard of care," it is wrong to perform placebo surgery on a patient because "surgeons do not perform surgery unless they judge it to be in the best interests of the patient." Miller argues, however, that this is not the right perspective from which to evaluate PCST. A randomized clinical trial is "not a form of personal medical therapy" but rather "a scientific tool for evaluating treatments." Miller notes that not just clinical trials but also a wide range of disease studies involve painful or potentially harmful interventions without any prospect of medical benefit to the participants. These risks to participants are generally judged acceptable when the risks are minimized and are not excessive and when the research stands to produce valuable knowledge.

> Clinical research, including treatment trials, would be impossible if it were held to the ethical standard of promoting the medical best interests of patients that governs therapeutic medicine. These ethically significant differences between clinical research and medical care—differences in purpose, methods, and justification of risks—imply that it is erroneous to hold that clinical research should be governed by the same ethical standards as apply to the practice of medicine. Sham surgery is not unethical just because it exposes patients to risks that are not compensated by medical benefits. Sham surgery as a control should be evaluated in terms of the ethical requirements proper to clinical research. (Miller 2003, 42)

This is a very striking claim—that research participants and patients inhabit two distinct ethical regimes and the exigencies of research demand that the research participants cannot be protected in the same way ordinary pa-tients are. One important difficulty with this idea is that people enrolled in studies are often both patient and research subjects and there is no clear de-marcation between research and treatment in many cases. Even if we could always categorize interventions as belonging to either research or clinical care, we may ask how is it that undertaking research confers on the re-searchers permission to take certain risks with the health of subjects that would be impermissible in the clinical context? The claim here is not that one consistent set of ethical principles has different practical implications in dif-ferent contexts, but that clinical care and medical research are properly reg-ulated according to different principles.

Miller's argument seems to be that because medical research sometimes requires doing things to participants that are not in their best interests, and because research can have valuable outcomes, such risks are therefore justi-fiable. Yet he accepts that in the context of clinical care, it is always wrong to act against a patient's best interest. It may well be true that it is practically impossible to conduct medical research without exposing subjects to risks without any expectation of a health benefit. However, this is not a *moral* ar-gument. Moral requirements are not proved on grounds of pragmatic neces-sity. Although it is not explicitly acknowledged, Miller's conception of the ethics of clinical research clearly has a utilitarian character.

> The ultimate question of risk-benefit assessment is whether the risks of sham arthroscopic surgery were justified by the anticipated scientific value of the study. We lack any objective tools for measuring research risk-benefit ratios. I contend that the relatively minor risks of the methodologically-indicated sham procedure were justifiable to answer the clinically important question of whether arthroscopic surgery is effective to treat pain associated with arthritis of the knee. This is a matter of judgment about which reasonable people might differ. (Miller 2003, 46)

Where Macklin opposes the "standards of research" with the "standards of ethics," Miller finds that there are two standards of ethics—one for re-search and one for clinical care. But we are not given any *principled* reason for the division between these domains. Why should the deontic constraints that regulate the doctor–patient relationship suddenly give out at the bound-ary between treatment and research? Why is the surgeon-qua-researcher en-titled to appeal to utilitarian justifications that are forbidden to the surgeon-qua-doctor?

At bottom, the reason why PCST is such a difficult and divisive issue is simply that this is a case where utilitarian and deontic principles conflict sharply. The dilemma cannot be resolved by simply ruling one or the other of these moral perspectives out of court. The utilitarian focuses on the com-parative magnitude of risks and benefits and abstracts away from their dis-tribution. From a utilitarian perspective, both the Parkinson's and knee surgery PCST described above were straightforwardly justifiable. In the case of the Parkinson's trial, the researchers, in their paper published before the trial, offered this rationale:

> The inclusion of a placebo group in our study of 36 subjects will permit us to establish whether the benefit observed to date can be attributed to an effect of treatment apart from a placebo effect. If fetal-tissue transplants are found to be safe and effective, thousands of patients with Parkinson's disease stand to benefit, and further research will be encouraged. If the transplants are found to be unsafe or ineffective, or if they offer nothing more than a placebo effect, hundreds or even thousands of patients will be spared the risks and financial burdens of an unproved operation. (Freeman et al. 1999)

Note that the trial is justified here in terms of benefits to future patients. When we consider, in addition, the flow-on effects of reallocating resources away from ineffective procedures, the utility sums clearly weigh in favor of such trials.

The deontic objection to this utilitarian argument concerns not the relative magnitude of risks and benefits but their distribution. Those who bear the risk of placebo surgery are not likely to be the direct beneficiaries of the knowledge obtained, and even where they do later benefit from improvements in treatment, other patients are effectively free-riders on the risks shouldered by the trial participants. There are various ways in which this kind of objection might be phrased. In Kantian terms, the subjects are treated as means rather than ends. In Rawlsian terms, fairness constraints are violated by making some individuals worse off for the benefit of others. The general form of the deontic objection to PCST is that such trials involve using patients in a way that is inconsistent with the duty to respect each individual patient's autonomy.

An unrestricted application of utilitarian reasoning would sanction research even where the subjects face substantial and certain harms, provided the research would lead to clearly greater benefits. For instance, imagine that one of the above trials was conducted without informing the subjects that the trial involved a placebo control. Such a trial would be quickly rejected by any ethics committee, although it might in fact be even better from a purely scientific perspective. Because utilitarianism does not give appropriate weight to the protection of individuals and their autonomy, contemporary standards in research ethics surround research subjects with various deontic protections. However, as Miller has observed, an absolute prohibition on harming some for the benefit of others would simply rule out a great part of medical research.

Clearly, research on humans is subject to *some* deontic constraints, and the debate around PCST is really about where to draw those limits. In practice, all the stress tends to fall on consent. Consent is the means of reconciling, or at least appearing to reconcile, these conflicting obligations. As long as the subject is informed of the risks and gives a valid consent, it appears that autonomy has been respected and researchers can go ahead and impose those risks. The moral acceptability of a PCST will hinge, then, on the _quality_ of consent from its subjects. What does consent to participation in a PCST need to be to do the moral work required of it?

In the case of surgical research, this tension is particularly acute. When surgical studies are designed according to good scientific methodology, with a randomized control, then it is uncomfortably clear that human subjects are going under the knife for research purposes. It is important to recognize here that surgical research has traditionally been conducted informally, and this is worse on _both_ consequentialist and patient-centered grounds. Informal surgical research has less evidential value and the progress of surgical practice goes more slowly and haphazardly than it otherwise might; and when patients undergo procedures unaware that some aspect of the procedure is experimental, then the status of their consent is questionable. PCST brings to the surface a moral dilemma that has hitherto been hidden, where surgeons have not been explicit with patients about surgery with a research component. The literature on the ethics of PCST has, for the most part, treated such trials in isolation and focused on the question of whether it is ever acceptable to perform a placebo operation. What has not been noticed is that the main arguments against PCST hold _a fortiori_ for informal surgical research, which is the most common mode of surgical research. If it is determined that PCST are ethically unacceptable, then this directly raises the question of whether any experimental surgery could be acceptable.

## EXPECTED VERSUS ACTUAL BENEFITS

To bring this point out, I want to draw attention to an important feature of the trials described above, which complicates the comparison with drug trials. Typically a drug trial compares a novel pharmaceutical against the standard therapy (or against placebo if there is none). The PCST conducted so far have aimed to assess procedures that were already in use. Before the Parkinson's PCST were conducted, fetal nigral tissue transplants were being performed by at least 17 centers. For arthroscopic lavage or débridement of the knee, Moseley and his colleagues (2002) report that more than 650,000 such procedures are performed annually in the United States. What this shows is that surgical procedures can become widespread without the kind of evidence supporting their efficacy that is required for the approval of new drugs. Indeed, there is a long list of surgical procedures that were once common and have since been discredited.

As Macklin puts it, the "chief reason" for disallowing PCST is that it is wrong to perform a surgical procedure that "has no expected benefit." So, that which justifies the risks of ordinary surgery is a reasonable expectation of benefit—which raises the question of when such expectations are reasonable. We might think that with common procedures the benefits are well established and the probability of a poor outcome or complications is accurately known. But the arthroscopic knee surgery example shows that this is not always true. With more radical procedures, such as fetal tissue transplants to repair brain damage, the uncertainty is greater, and centers were reporting a success rate which, it turned out, could not be reproduced in a rigorous, randomized control trial. For patients who received the placebo operation, it seems clear that no benefit could be reasonably expected from a "pretend" operation. But was there a *reasonable* expectation of benefit for the patients who received the transplants, or for the patients who underwent this procedure in other clinics?

Expectations are probabilistic—an operation may offer a high or a low chance of success. It is easy for expectations to be inflated by hope. What differentiates wishful thinking from a reasonable expectation of benefit is that there is an evidence base supporting the judgment that a beneficial outcome is probable. Where the evidence is missing or unreliable, where patients give consent with misleading or no information about the actual probability of benefits and harms, we cannot say that there is a reasonable expectation of benefit. In the Parkinson's PCST, the transplant recipients as a group did not show better than a placebo effect, and some experienced serious complications. This means that those who received the placebo operation had roughly the same chance of benefit and a much lower chance of harm than those who received the transplant. It then seems odd to say that it was only the placebo procedures that were wrong because they had no expected benefit. Correct expectations as to the probability of benefit and harm would have offered even less comfort to those subjects who had the trial procedure.

Patients and surgeons may subjectively expect that a procedure will work, but subjective expectations can be sadly mistaken and the mere psychological state of expecting a benefit does not of itself justify running a serious risk. What is required is that benefits are *reasonably* expected, meaning the expectations are supported by good evidence. The very purpose of PCST is to generate good evidence about the efficacy of procedures in cases where it is lacking. Where reliable evidence of safety and efficacy is not available for a surgical procedure, there are no persuasive reasons to expect a benefit from undergoing that procedure. Imagine that you had to participate in a PCST, but you were allowed to choose whether you receive the trial procedure or the placebo operation. If you decided on expected utility alone, the rational choice would actually be to join the placebo group: You don't have good reason to expect the experimental procedure to work, and you know that you are far less likely to be harmed in the placebo arm. You could then choose the experimental procedure later, if and when it is proven effective.

If surgery is only justified by a sound expectation of net benefit, then it is not only placebo surgery that fails to meet that standard. Now we see why

PCST presents a deeper dilemma than its critics have realized. If we accept the principal argument against PCST, then, on the same grounds, we should object even more strenuously to speculative procedures and informal surgical research. Yet a ban on PCST means that surgical research remains confined to methods that are morally worse, and ineffective procedures that would be exposed by a PCST may remain in use.

## THE CONSENT OF THE DESPERATE

When important research unavoidably requires that participants are put at risk, the moral acceptability of that research depends heavily on the quality of consent obtained. The Parkinson's PCST was rightly criticized in this regard because the consent of subjects was likely to be compromised by the "therapeutic misconception." The therapeutic misconception is a well-documented problem with patients entering drug trials, particularly phase 1 trials for cancer and other terminal conditions. Phase 1 drug trials are primarily intended to determine toxicity and dosage limits and are not designed to yield a therapeutic benefit for the enrolled subjects. Participation in such a trial is really an altruistic act of loaning one's body to medical science. Nevertheless, there is considerable evidence that many patients enroll in such trials in hope of getting better. In a paper on the therapeutic misconception in phase 1 cancer trials, Matthew Miller (2000) writes:

> Given that the remission rate is less than 1 percent and that the rate of death due to drug toxicity is comparable, few would claim any aggregate survival advantage for participants. In fact, consent documents state that Phase 1 cancer trials are primarily toxicity studies and that response is neither intended nor expected. Yet patients enrolled in these trials overwhelmingly cite hope of physical benefit (rarely altruism) as their primary motivation for enrolling.

How blameworthy researchers are in this regard is a difficult question. Trial subjects who have the therapeutic misconception are being exploited. Yet the psychology of the doctor–patient relationship makes it difficult for doctors to disabuse very sick patients of whatever slim hopes they have. Clearly though, the therapeutic misconception fatally compromises patient consent. Recall that participants in the Parkinson's PCST were told that if they received the placebo, and the procedure proved effective, they would be offered the procedure. Such an offer implicitly invites candidates to believe that enrolling in the trial might offer a route to recovery.

Macklin (1999) cites reports of patient anger in the Parkinson's trial when placebo recipients were told that, because of safety considerations, the real procedure would not be offered. She asks if it is overly paternalistic to protect research subjects from risks they seem willing to accept, and suggests, "The emphasis today on respect for the autonomy of patients and research subjects creates a reluctance to question whether their choices are fully rational." Macklin appears to argue that the obstacles to informed consent are too great in this case and patients should not be offered such a choice.

Franklin Miller accepts that the therapeutic misconception may have been present in the Parkinson's trial, but contends that this result cannot be generalized to all PCST. He contends that the patients in the arthroscopic surgery trial were not "vulnerable" because, although arthritis is painful, "it is not associated with impaired decision-making capacity" (2003, 46).

Perhaps "autonomy" has become a buzzword often used too carelessly to sanction irrational patient choices. Properly understood, respect for autonomy actually demands that we test the rationality of questionable choices and make greater efforts to help patients understand the salient facts. Irrationality is commonplace and sick people are especially prone to it, but that fact does not warrant a pessimistic retreat to paternalism. Well-designed PCST can yield information of great value. The problem with PCST is that participants are asked to submit to risks without a compensating expectation of benefit to their health. It is not irrational for a patient to believe that contributing to medical knowledge or helping future sufferers of his condition is sufficient reason to participate in a surgical trial.

PCST are not inherently or necessarily unethical, but we must be sure that participants understand that therapeutic benefit is not the primary goal of the trial and that there is a high chance that they will get no health benefit. Ethics committees reviewing proposed PCST need to be satisfied that there is adequate testing to ensure that participant consent is not motivated by an unfounded hope of improved health. We should expect that this will make it harder to find volunteers, but if that is the price of adequate consent then so be it.

I will conclude by pointing out that there is one obvious way to ameliorate the problem of uncompensated harm, and that is to compensate. If participants volunteering for surgical research suffer complications, then they should receive not just treatment but also some monetary compensation for that suffering. Compensating for adverse outcomes is not the same as paying participants and cannot reasonably be construed as an inducement. My proposal is that fair compensatory payouts for various complications be determined in advance and that this information be part of the informed consent process. I believe this would help potential volunteers to appreciate the reality and relative seriousness of the risks they are being asked to accept. Such a scheme would require insurance coverage, which would increase the cost of trials. If it is objected that this would make surgical trials too costly, that is equivalent to an admission that the funding of such research depends on unfair cost shifting onto trial subjects. The case of PCST offers a stark illustration of how the costs of medical progress are disproportionately borne by research subjects. If we are serious about eliminating exploitation in medical research, then patients who are harmed in such studies must be compensated.

## NOTE

1. The authors refer to statistics showing that more than 650,000 such procedures are performed annually in the United States, costing approximately $5,000 each.

## REFERENCES

Albin, R. L. 2002. Sham surgery controls: Intracerebral grafting of fetal tissue for Parkinson's disease and proposed criteria for use of sham surgery controls. *Journal of Medical Ethics* 28 (5): 322–25.

Beecher, Henry K. 1961. Surgery as placebo: A quantitative study of bias. *Journal of the American Medical Association* 176 (13): 1102–07.

Clark, Peter A. 2002. Placebo surgery for Parkinson's Disease: Do the benefits outweigh the risks? *Journal of Law, Medicine and Ethics* 30 (1): 58–68.

Fletcher, John C. 2003. Sham neurosurgery in Parkinson's disease: Ethical at the time. *American Journal of Bioethics* 3 (4): 54–56.

Freed, Curt R., Paul E. Greene, Robert E. Breeze, Wei-Yann Tsai, William DuMouchel, Richard Kao, Sandra Dillon, Howard Winfield, Sharon Culver, John Q. Trojanowski, David Eidelberg, and Stanley Fahn. 2001. Transplantation of embryonic dopamine neurons for severe Parkinson's disease. *New England Journal of Medicine* 344 (10): 710–19.

Freeman, Thomas B., Dorothy E. Vawter, Paul E. Leaverton, James H. Godbold, Robert A. Hauser, Christopher G. Goetz, and C. Warren Olanow. 1999. Use of placebo surgery in controlled trials of a cellular-based therapy for Parkinson's disease. *New England Journal of Medicine* 341 (13): 988–92.

Macklin, Ruth. 1999. The ethical problems with sham surgery in clinical research. *New England Journal of Medicine* 341 (13): 992–96.

Miller, Franklin G. 2003. Sham surgery: An ethical analysis. *American Journal of Bioethics* 3 (4): 41–48.

Miller, Matthew. 2000. Phase 1 cancer trials: A collusion of misunderstanding. *Hastings Center Report* 30 (4): 34–42.

Moseley, J. Bruce, Kimberly O'Malley, Nancy J. Petersen, Terri J. Menke, Baruch A. Brody, David H. Kuykendall, John C. Hollingsworth, Carol M. Ashton, and Nelda P. Wray. 2002. A controlled trial of arthroscopic surgery for osteoarthritis of the knee. *New England Journal of Medicine* 347 (2): 81–88.

Reitsma, Angelique M., and Jonathan D. Moreno. 2002. Ethical regulations for innovative surgery: The last frontier? *Journal of the American College of Surgeons* 194 (6): 792–801.

———. 2003. Surgical research, an elusive entity. *American Journal of Bioethics* 3 (4): 49–50.

# 13

# Sham Surgery
# and Reasonable Risks

*Alex John London*

One of the most fundamental tensions within clinical research arises from the need to balance the goal of advancing the frontiers of science in order to improve the standard of care available to future persons with the goal of responding with diligence and compassion to the important interests and health needs of the research participants who make such progress possible (Jonas 1969; see also London 2003). Although this tension pervades clinical research, it is particularly salient in the debate over the use of placebo controls in clinical trials.[1] Recently however, the already contentious debate about the conditions under which it is permissible to include a placebo arm in a clinical trial has been further complicated by several clinical trials in which participants have been randomized to a sham-surgery control.

To many critics, sham-surgery controls differ in morally significant ways from traditional placebo controls (Macklin 1999; see also London and Kadane 2002). Generally speaking, traditional placebo controls are inert substances that are chosen precisely because of their causal inefficacy. The primary worry associated with the use of such substances are the opportunity costs that participants may incur from being randomized to them. These opportunity costs are cause for ethical concern, for example, when randomizing participants with a particular medical condition to a placebo deprives them of the opportunity to access an alternative treatment modality that is otherwise available for their condition. While opportunity costs remain a concern in the case of sham-surgery controls, the latter also raise additional concerns because the so-called placebo or sham surgeries often involve actual surgical interventions that carry their own special risks and burdens. Unlike the relatively benign profile of the traditional, inert placebo, sham-surgery controls may require recipients to undergo invasive and burdensome surgical procedures whose purpose is not to treat the recipient but simply to maintain the methodological rigor of the study. The affirmative risks and burdens that may be associated with such procedures have marked out sham-surgery controls for special scrutiny and concern (Dekkers and Boer 2001; Clark 2002; London and Kadane 2002; Weijer 2002).

However, recent interest in utilizing sham-surgery controls has been motivated, in large part, by an increased desire to subject surgical procedures to what is viewed as the gold-standard for clinical research, the randomized, double-blind, placebo-controlled trial. Unlike pharmaceuticals or implantable medical devices, surgical procedures are largely free from regulatory oversight (Reitsma and Moreno 2002; Bower 2003). Those who defend the use of sham-surgery controls, therefore, emphasize the desirability of requiring rigorous evidence of efficacy for surgical procedures (Freeman et al. 1999; Horng and Miller 2002; Miller 2003). In particular, they claim that a sham-surgery control is necessary in order to effectuate a blinded study in which the first-person experience of participants in each trial arm is comparable. Moreover, proponents of sham-surgical controls are quick to point out that there are many elements of clinical trials that subject participants to risks or burdens without the prospect of direct personal benefit. That is, proponents argue that from an analytical point of view a sham-surgery control is no different from the extra blood draws, spinal taps, or other diagnostic procedures to which subjects are routinely subjected within the context of a well-designed clinical trial but which would not be administered in the context of routine clinical practice.

Perhaps somewhat ironically, therefore, one of the central issues in the debate about the ethics of sham-surgery controls is whether these practices even raise special concerns over and above those that routinely arise in the evaluation of clinical research. While some view them as largely contiguous with existing methods and practices in clinical research, others see them as practices that require special justification or which should be prohibited outright. In either case, these disagreements reflect the significant lack of consensus within research ethics about the moral status of sham-surgery controls.

In the discussion that follows, I argue that even if the ethical issues that are associated with these practices are not qualitatively different from standard ethical issues that arise in the course of clinical research, the ethical issues that these practices do raise are nevertheless particularly important and warrant placing the burden of proof on researchers to show that the use of such a design in a particular case is ethically permissible. On a deeper level, however, I argue that the lack of consensus about the moral status of sham-surgery controls reflects a more profound conflict within the research ethics community about the nature and the extent of the risks to which it is permissible to subject research participants. In order to clarify the ethical issues that are raised by the use of sham-surgery controls, as well and to illustrate this deeper conflict within the research ethics community, I begin with a brief portrait of three sham-surgery-controlled clinical trials. I then examine several proposed standards for evaluating trials of this kind and argue that none is entirely adequate. Finally, I conclude with a proposal that clinical research must conform to a particular principle of equal respect and argue that sham-surgery controls should be permitted only in cases where they are consistent with such a principle.

## A TALE OF THREE SHAM SURGERIES

### Case 1. Arthroscopic Surgery for Osteoarthritis of the Knee

Each year roughly 650,000 arthroscopic débridement or lavage procedures are performed as a treatment for osteoarthritis of the knee (Moseley et al. 2002). At roughly $5,000 per procedure, the annual cost of these procedures is about $3.25 billion. In 2002 Moseley and colleagues reported the results of a sham-surgery-controlled, double-blind, randomized clinical trial of arthroscopic surgery for osteoarthritis of the knee. In this study, a total of 180 patients with osteoarthritis of the knee were randomized to receive either arthroscopic débridement, arthroscopic lavage, or "placebo surgery." Those who were randomized to the sham-surgery control were given a short-acting intravenous tranquilizer and an opioid while members of the surgical team simulated a standard arthroscopic débridement procedure. In other words, subjects were conscious in the operating theater, where their knees were draped and prepped and the surgical team manipulated both the subject's knee and the medical instruments as though standard operations were being performed. In actuality, subjects received only a one-centimeter incision in their skin; no instruments were inserted into the opening. Each group received comparable postoperative care consisting of walking aids, a graduated exercise program, and analgesics. Each subject was followed for two years and the primary end point of the study was pain, although functionality was a secondary efficacy endpoint.

### Case 2. Fetal Nigral Cell Transplants for Parkinson's Disease

Parkinson's disease is a degenerative neurological disorder characterized by a loss of dopaminergic neurons in the basal ganglia of the brain, producing tremors, muscle rigidity, and abnormal movements. The standard treatment, oral doses of the dopamine precursor Levodopa, reverses these symptoms in most patients, but over time its effects tend to wear off and its side-effect profile increases. In 1999 Freeman and colleagues reported the results of a double-blind, randomized, sham-surgery-controlled trial in which 36 subjects were randomized to one of three arms, two receiving bilateral fetal nigral transplantation and one receiving bilateral placebo surgery. Throughout the study, all subjects continued to receive standard medical therapy. Just as members of the first two arms underwent two surgical procedures, the control group received two placebo surgical procedures that were designed "to provide an equivalent experience for the subjects and their family members" (Freeman et al. 1999). Each placebo procedure involved the placement of a stereotactic frame—a frame attached to the cranium with surgical screws, which allows for accurate location of targeted areas in the brain—a magnetic resonance imaging (MRI) scan, a positron-emission tomography (PET) scan, the administration of general anesthesia, and the drilling of two dime-sized burr holes into the skull through scalp incisions. In the control group, the burr holes did not penetrate the dura and no material was injected into the brain. All subjects, however, received intravenous antibiotics and cyclosporine for six months after surgery.

## Case 3. Trial of Glial Cell Line–Derived Neurotrophic Factors (GDNF) for Parkinson's Disease

In 2003, Nutt and colleagues reported the results of a randomized, double-blind, placebo-controlled trial of GDNF for Parkinson's disease. This phase 1–2 trial was designed to assess the safety, tolerability, and biological activity of GDNF—a peptide that had been shown to promote the survival of dopamine neurons in animal models—in subjects with moderately advanced Parkinson's disease. Its primary end points for safety and tolerability were adverse events, vital signs, and various laboratory measures, and the trial was not powered to detect specific changes in any efficacy measure. In this trial, each of the 80 enrolled subjects received an implanted intracerebroventricular (ICV) cannula connected to an access port that was implanted under their scalp. In other words, each subject was placed into a stereotactic frame and had an opening drilled through their skull into which a small flexible tube was inserted so that either the study material or a placebo could be delivered to the subject's brain. Subjects were then randomized to receive either escalating doses of ICV GDNF or an ICV placebo for a period of six to eight months.

## CONFLICTING EVALUATIONS

The recent debate over the use of sham-surgery controls has focused, in large part, on central ethical issues that are spelled out in the U.S. code of federal regulations which institutional review boards (IRBs) in the United States are required to use in evaluating particular research initiatives. These regulations require IRBs to ensure that:

1. Risks to subjects are minimized: (i) by using procedures which are consistent with sound research design and which do not unnecessarily expose subjects to risk, and (ii) whenever appropriate, by using procedures already being performed on the subjects for diagnostic or treatment purposes.
2. Risks to subjects are reasonable in relation to anticipated benefits, if any, to subjects, and the importance of the knowledge that may reasonably be expected to result. In evaluating risks and benefits, the IRB should consider only those risks and benefits that may result from the research (as distinguished from risks and benefits of therapies subjects would receive even if not participating in the research). The IRB should not consider possible long-range effects of applying knowledge gained in the research (for example, possible effects of the research on public policy) as among those research risks that fall within the purview of its responsibility.[2]

Although each side of this debate couches its ethical analysis in the language that is laid out in the above guidelines, each arrives at very different views about some of the above cases. The reason for this conflict in assessments lies in the fact that each side ultimately embraces significantly different views about the larger social role of clinical research and the scope and limits of what it is permissible to ask of research subjects.

For example, the arguments offered by Freeman and colleagues to defend their use of a sham-surgery control in case 2 are emblematic of the approach of those who defend the use of sham-surgery controls more generally. First, Freeman and colleagues argue for the methodological necessity of including a sham-surgery control in their trial. In particular, they claim that it is an indispensable component of a trial that is designed to answer their chosen research question: is fetal-tissue transplantation a safe and effective treatment for Parkinson's disease and, if so, are the observed benefits the result of the fetal-tissue transplant or of some associated placebo effect? Second, they then argue that, against this methodological background, "the risks to participants are reasonable and have been minimized as far as possible" (Freeman et al. 1999, 991). In particular, members of the control group continue to receive standard medical therapy for Parkinson's disease, a partial burr hole is used instead of penetrating the dura, no material is inserted in the brains of subjects, and renal function is monitored to detect adverse reactions to cyclosporine.

The claim of Freeman and colleagues that the risks to the control group have been minimized in their trial takes the risks that are associated with the active arm as the proper baseline of evaluation. Whereas the holes in the heads of subjects in the active arm penetrate the dura, those of control arm do not. Whereas subjects in the active arm have material inserted into their brains, members of the control group do not. Relative to this baseline, the risks to members of the control group have been minimized as far as is consistent with maintaining the integrity of a sound clinical trial design. Although sham-surgery controls may subject participants to risks and burdens that are not compensated for by any prospect of direct therapeutic benefit, this approach claims that their use does not *unnecessarily* expose subjects to risk as long as those risks and burdens have been minimized as far as is consistent with a sound trial design.

In contrast, critics of sham-surgery controls are reluctant to use the risks that are associated with the intervention in the active arm as the baseline for determining whether the risks to members of the control group have been minimized. For example, in her evaluation of case 2, Ruth Macklin argues that "the question of how great the risks of sham surgery are in any particular trial is distinct from the question of whether a surgical intervention carries risks of harm that are greater than those associated with no surgical intervention" (1999, 993). Here, Macklin appears to be asserting that the proper baseline against which the risks to members of the control group should be evaluated is the situation in which they are not subjected to any surgical procedure at all. In other words, the proper baseline in this particular case would be the provision of their standard medical therapy and a more traditional, inert placebo. It is against this background assumption that Macklin asserts that "it is undeniable that performing surgery in research subjects that has no potential therapeutic benefit fails to minimize the risks of harm" (993).

On this particular issue, therefore, the difference between critics and proponents of sham-surgery controls boils down to the more fundamental question of how to set the proper baseline against which the risks to subjects in the control group are evaluated. Each of the above proposals has one distinct virtue: operational clarity. That is, Macklin and Freeman and colleagues each provide clear, though very different, standards for determining the limits of the risks to which members of the sham-surgery arm of a trial may permissibly be exposed. Moreover, each of their proposed standards yields a determinate evaluation of each of the three cases described above. Despite this singular virtue, however, each position appears to err in opposite directions. Whereas Macklin's position is overly conservative, the approach of Freeman and colleagues is overly permissive.

The conservative nature of Macklin's position can be illustrated by consideration of case 1. Proponents have been quick to argue that the sort of sweeping condemnation of sham surgery controls that results from Macklin's position would rule out as unethical the sham-surgery control that Moseley and colleagues employed in this study (Miller 2003, 45–46). After all, subjects in the control arm received a tranquilizer, an opioid, and one-centimeter incisions in the skin of their knees. These risks are greater than the baseline situation of not receiving any surgery at all and would therefore be ruled out as ethically impermissible in Macklin's view. In fact, it looks like Macklin's view would rule out a similar trial design in which subjects were spared the risks associated with the tranquilizer and the opioid but were still subjected to one-centimeter skin incisions in their knees. To critics, this result reduces such a rigid and conservative position to absurdity.

In contrast, the approach endorsed by Freeman and colleagues would justify not only each of three cases described above but also the use of even the most invasive and burdensome sham-surgery controls. The permissiveness of this approach results from two factors (London and Kadane 2002). First, because it evaluates the risks to subjects in the control arm against the baseline of the risks to which subjects are exposed in the active arm or arms, this approach would permit extremely invasive and burdensome sham-surgery controls so long as those controls had fewer risks and burdens than the intervention in the active arm. If, for instance, the active arm were a new coronary surgery, this approach would permit a sham-surgery control in which the body cavity of subjects is opened but no additional intervention is performed.

Such a control would have to be justified, of course, as having reduced the risks as far as possible consistent with the integrity of the trial design. Notice, however, that the integrity of a trial design relates to its ability to generate the information necessary to answer the particular question that the trial is designed to answer. The second feature of this approach that makes it overly permissive is that it provides few resources, if any, for assessments of whether the question that the trial is designed to answer is an appropriate or acceptable question to pursue at that time. The level to which the risks to subjects in the sham-surgery arm must be reduced is a direct product of the specific question that the researchers have chosen to pursue. If, as in case 3, researchers want to distinguish the clinical effects of the implanted material from the effects of the general surgical procedure that accompanies that intervention, they would be largely free to subject members of the control group to highly invasive and burdensome sham-surgical procedures in order to do so. Although such information may always be of interest from a purely scientific point of view, such fastidiousness may be unnecessary from a more pragmatic or clinically oriented point of view. The approach under question, however, lacks the internal resources to draw such lines in a clear and principled way.

Worries of the latter sort are particularly salient in case 3 above. Although intracerebroventricular administration of GDNF had shown promising results in rodent and monkey models of Parkinson's disease, its tolerability, safety, and effectiveness in humans had not been established. The purpose of the study by Nutt and colleagues was to assess the safety, tolerability, and biological activity of ICV GDNF in patients with advanced Parkinson's. The placebo-controlled design was used to maintain the double-blinded standard and to hold constant changes in the condition of recipients that might be due to the ICV catheter and the administration of a substance into the brain, thereby more accurately isolating effects specifically related to the GDNF itself. This particularly intrusive placebo control therefore enabled the researchers to isolate adverse events that were associated with the administration of GDNF from those associated with the surgical elements of the procedure itself.

In this case, serious questions can be raised about the appropriateness of trying to answer this explanatory question rather than assessing the safety and tolerability of ICV administration of GDNF and *all that it entails* relative to the baseline condition of subjects with advanced Parkinson's disease receiving a more benign placebo—one that involved more sham and less surgery. After all, the various components of this intervention cannot be separated in practice; one cannot administer GDNF to the brain of a patient without creating a pathway of access through the skull. From a clinical standpoint, therefore, concerns about safety and tolerability do not apply simply to the GDNF and its effects on the brain. Rather they encompass all necessary elements of the procedure, including the ICV cannula and access port. Even if we grant the claim that Nutt and colleagues reduced the risks to study participants as far as possible, consistent with the integrity of their preferred trial design, it is questionable whether it was appropriate at the time to ask the particular research question that required such a fastidious and burdensome trial design.

Prospective worries of this sort appear to be borne out by the results of this particular study. The trial was terminated after a total of 50 participants, 12 of whom were randomized to the placebo, completed the double-blind portion of the study. With respect to effects on measures relating to parkinsonism, the placebo weakly dominated the active intervention, meaning that there were either no significant differences between the placebo and the active agent or the measured difference favored the placebo. Similar results were obtained on measures of safety and tolerability. Whereas 92 percent of subjects randomized to placebo suffered treatment-associated adverse effects, adverse effects were reported by 100 percent of subjects who received the active agent. Adverse effects that related to the implanted cannula and access port included headache (25 percent of the placebo group, 71 percent of the active group) and nausea (25 percent of the placebo group, 87 percent of the active group), with serious adverse events including an extended hospitalization of a patient due to difficulties removing the device and a bacterial colonization of the access port in another patient whose port therefore had to be removed and reimplanted.

Although the nature of the sham-surgery in case 3 is significantly more burdensome than the one employed in case 2, similar reservations have been articulated in the latter case as well (London and Kadane 2002). In both cases, legitimate questions arise about the permissibility of employing the burdensome methods necessary to explain which effects measured in the trial are associated with which elements of the experimental intervention before one has addressed the more pragmatic issue of whether or not the experimental procedure as a whole has effects that make it attractive from a clinical point of view.

## UNCERTAINTY ABOUT REASONABLE RISKS

Not all proponents of sham-surgery controls are wedded to the framework proposed by Freeman and colleagues. Miller, for example, has argued that

Macklin's position is overly restrictive largely on the grounds that it misconstrues the requirements of the federal regulations (Miller 2003, 45–46). After all, although condition 2 in the above-cited regulations requires that risks must be reasonable in relation to the benefits subjects may receive from participating in the research, it is also clear that subjects need not themselves receive any such benefit for the research to be acceptable. What condition 2 actually requires in this regard is an evaluation of the reasonableness of the risks posed to participants in relation to the importance of the knowledge that may result from the research (Weijer 2000).

Miller argues that in case 1, the risks associated with the sham-surgery control were justified in light of the methodological rigor of the trial design and the importance of the research question. After all, the resources that are expended each year on the procedures being studied are far from inconsequential and the surgical procedure itself is far from risk free. Moreover, although a research initiative must be judged as ethical or unethical at its inception, Miller claims that the merits of their position are borne out by the actual results of the trial. At the conclusion of the study, Moseley and colleagues reported that there was no point at which recipients of either of the active interventions reported less pain or better functionality than recipients of the sham-surgery control. In fact, recipients of actual débridement had poorer objective measures of walking and stair climbing at two weeks and one year, and they showed a trend toward worse functioning at two years than did recipients of the sham-surgery control. The research that generated these significant findings, they emphasize, would have been prohibited under Macklin's guidelines.

Although Miller's approach to assessing the risks to which it is permissible to subject research participants is more permissive than the one articulated by Macklin, it lacks the operational clarity that is a hallmark of her approach as well as the one endorsed by Freeman and colleagues. In particular, neither Miller's approach nor the federal regulations from which it is derived provide an account of (1) what constitutes "the importance of the knowledge that may reasonably be expected to result" from a particular research initiative or (2) how this might be measured. The practical result of this absence of operational clarity is that the boundaries of what different deliberators might accept as a measure of the importance of such knowledge is set only by the limits of the imaginations of the various deliberating agents (London and Kadane 2003). Moreover, even if a set of agents share the same view on this issue, neither Miller nor the federal regulations provide a clear standard for determining the permissible limits of the risks to which research subjects may be subjected in *exchange for such gains in knowledge*—however they are understood.

On this point, at least, Miller is clear: he holds that "the ultimate question of risk-assessment" is whether the risks of sham surgery are justified by the anticipated scientific value of the study, and says that, ultimately, "we lack any objective tools for measuring research risk–benefit ratios" (Miller 2003,

46). However, if we remain content with such a state of affairs, then we must also be prepared to accept the reality that the discrepancies between proponents such as Miller and critics like Macklin simply boil down to different intuitions about whether the risks of sham-surgery controls are in some inchoate sense "worth it" (Kim 2003). Such an approach provides little guidance about how to bring reasoned resolution to the significant range of unresolved conflicts that exists when deliberators who apply a shared set of standards are incapable of reaching a consensus on the moral standing of a particular research initiative. In the worst case, the field would simply be divided by conflicting intuitions about how to proceed here as well. In Macklin's opinion, for example, when reasonable people disagree about the risks that subjects bear in sham-surgery-controlled clinical trials, the default position should be a conservative approach to the use of such practices. In contrast, proponents of sham-surgery controls may incline more toward a position that allows methodologically rigorous clinical research to go forward unless there is a social consensus that it would be unethical to do so.

While Miller seems to think that his approach would be less permissive than the one I am attributing to Freeman and colleagues, it is unclear whether this would necessarily be so. Because the judgments that Miller's view requires deliberators to make are largely intuitive, and because the framework provides little operational guidance about how to make such judgments, it is not clear that it would help well-intentioned deliberators form a considered opinion about more controversial cases such as case 2 or case 3. Nor is it clear that Miller's approach is inconsistent with that of Freeman and colleagues. In fact, it seems clear that *both* Macklin and Freeman and colleagues could reasonably argue that their positions should be understood as presuming Miller's general framework in which risks to subjects are balanced against gains in knowledge. That is, both could argue that they are presenting operationally clear, concrete proposals regarding *how to determine* whether the risks to subjects are permissible in light of the potential benefits to science.[3]

The fact that views as disparate as those of Macklin and Freeman and colleagues can be presented under the rubric of ensuring the reasonability of risks provides a powerful illustration of the uncertainty surrounding the operational content of this general requirement. It also illustrates how relatively local skirmishes over the ethics of sham-surgery controls reflect these more fundamental uncertainties. This connection helps to explain my contention that sham-surgery controls raise issues of special ethical significance, even if these issues are not qualitatively different from those that are faced in trials that are not sham-surgery controlled. Persistent uncertainties about sham-surgery controls are symptomatic of a larger uncertainty in the field concerning the limits of the risks to which trial participants may permissibly be subjected. Although sham-surgery controls highlight in a particularly dramatic fashion the extent to which the demands of science may be at odds with the interests of trial participants, other elements of clinical trials frequently raise similar issues. This general problem is of fundamental moral importance because it deals with the extent to which the interests of trial participants can be compromised or sacrificed for the good of future persons. Any effort to forge a consensus about the ethical use of sham-surgery controls, therefore, will have to confront ambiguities surrounding these larger issues explicitly and in a principled manner.

## FAIRNESS TO EQUALITY: A TENTATIVE PROPOSAL

I suggested above that the central difference between Macklin and Freeman and colleagues lies in the different baselines they use to evaluate the risks in a clinical trial. Although the difficulties associated with each of their approaches stem from limitations in the specific baselines they adopt, the fact that each articulates such a clear baseline for making such judgments gives their views an operational clarity that is missing in the Common Rule. Any view that hopes to overcome these limitations in a way that preserves this kind of operational clarity will have to provide a clear answer to each of the following questions (London 2005).

1. How should the concept of "reasonable risk" be understood?
2. What are the criteria or practical markers that can be used in order to delineate in an operationally useful way the parameters or boundaries that separate reasonable from excessive risks?
3. What are the tests or mechanisms that deliberators can use in order to determine whether or not these operational criteria have been met in any particular case?

In this section I will outline tentative answers to each of these questions and show how the resulting framework would discriminate between the cases described above.

To begin with, it is not sufficient to link the reasonableness of a risk simply to the importance of the prospective benefits of research. One must go further and specify whether or not, for the individual trial subject, there is a threshold beyond which risks cannot be outweighed by benefits in science. As a starting point, therefore, we should consider what reasonable limitations there should be on the risks that it is permissible for society to allow its clinical researchers to offer to prospective trial participants. Put slightly differently, if the institution of clinical research is going to function as part of a social division of labor that is justifiable to the members of the community whose interests it is supposed to serve, then what are the limits of the risks that it may offer to prospective participants while serving this function?

Each member of society can recognize that all have a fundamental interest in ensuring that the basic social structures of their community function to safeguard their most basic human interests. In this context, "basic interests" refers to the set of interests that each individual community member shares with all other community members in being able to cultivate and exercise their rudimentary intellectual, affective, and social capacities in the pursuit of a meaningful life plan. Basic interests should be distinguished from what I will call "personal interests," in that the latter are interests that individuals form as the result of pursuing a particular set of goals or plans and as the result of exercising the set of basic interests that make these ends and activities possible (London 2003). In liberal democratic communities, individuals may differ widely in their personal interests and may reasonably disagree about the value or significance of the personal interests of their fellow citizens. Nevertheless, each is capable of recognizing that all share a set of basic interests in being able to cultivate and exercise the rudimentary intellectual, affective, and social capacities that make it possible for them to form, pursue, and revise their respective personal interests.[4]

Because basic interests can be profoundly restricted or defeated by sickness and disease, each can recognize a reason to support medical research as a social institution insofar as it strives to advance the state of medical science and therefore the standard of care that is available to community members. As one element within a larger social division of labor that must be justifiable to the members of the community whose basic interests it is supposed to serve, clinical research must pursue its goal of advancing the interests of future patients in a way that is consistent with an equal regard for the basic interests of the present persons whose participation makes those results possible.

The requirement to respect the basic interests of both present participants and future beneficiaries supports the following proposal for a definition of *reasonable risk*.

> ***Concept of Reasonable Risk:*** Reasonable risks are those that are necessary in order to generate important scientific information and that are consistent with an equal regard for the basic interests of study participants and the members of the larger community whose interests that research is intended to serve.

The requirement that risks be consistent with an equal regard for the basic interests of study participants and members of the larger community is intended to reflect the idea that even if the beneficiaries of the research enterprise can cite a moral imperative to carry out research as part of an effort to help to safeguard their basic interests, such an imperative cannot legitimate requiring others to sacrifice or to forfeit their basic interests in the process.[5] In other words, the same concern to advance the interests of future patients that underwrites the research enterprise as a social institution cannot be withheld from present, prospective research participants.

Operational criteria can be generated for this conception of reasonable risk by considering how the basic interests of community members are safeguarded and advanced by the larger social division of labor. For the kinds of cases we have been considering here, where the basic interests of persons are threatened or restricted by sickness, injury, or disease, this job falls, in large part, to the health care system. This suggests adopting the following operational criterion for determining whether efforts to advance the standard of care for future patients show an equal regard for research participants and nonparticipants.

> ***Operational Criterion:*** Within the research context, equal regard for the basic interests of participants and nonparticipants requires that the basic interests of participants be protected and advanced in a way that does not fall below the threshold of competent medical care.

It is important to note several features of this operational criterion. First, its scope is limited to the basic interests of participants for two primary reasons: (1) It is supposed to delineate the level of risk that it is permissible to *offer* to prospective participants; participants are then free to decide for themselves whether the risks that remain in a trial that meets this standard are acceptable in light of their particular personal interests. (2) The focus on basic interests reflects the normative claim that it is permissible to ask individual community members to alter, risk, or even to sacrifice some of their *personal interests* as part of an effort to advance or secure the *basic interests* of others. It is not, however, permissible to ask community members to sacrifice their basic interests in order to advance or safeguard the personal interests of others.

Another significant feature of the stated operational criterion is that several reasons underwrite using the threshold of competent medical care as a practical standard for determining whether the level of protection and care that a research initiative provides is consistent with an equal regard for the basic interests of participants and nonparticipants: (1) Competent medical care represents the socially enforceable standard of professional knowledge, skill, and ability that community members have a legitimate claim to receive when they access the medical system; although some clinicians may rise above the rest in terms of various professional excellences, competent medical care denotes the level of care that the medical profession is accountable for providing on a uniform basis. (2) Competent medical care refers to the use of practices, procedures, and methods that have a reasonable likelihood of success; in this respect, it serves as an indicator of what expert medical professionals believe is a causally efficacious means of effectuating desired clinical goals.

It is often the case that competent medical care does not provide a single, well-ordered standard of care for dealing with particular medical conditions. The boundaries of competent care often include a variety of alternative approaches for dealing with a particular condition. This may be the result of different traditions of practice that adopt different methods for dealing with a particular condition. It can also result when there is uncertainty within the expert medical community about what constitutes the optimal method of dealing with a condition generally or for treating specific individual patients with that particular medical condition.

The fact that there is often no single, well-ordered standard of competent medical care can thus be used to create a practical test for assessing whether particular research initiatives are acceptable in light of the operational criterion articulated above.

> *Practical Test:* For each individual within a particular clinical trial, the care and protection that is provided to that individual's basic interests falls within the threshold of competent medical care when it represents an admissible intervention in light of either uncertainty in the form of agnosticism or conflict in the expert medical community about the relative net therapeutic advantage of that package of care in comparison to alternative packages that are available either within the trial itself or within the context of clinical care.

This practical test is similar to what Freedman (1987) referred to as "clinical equipoise," although there are some important differences.[6] For example, clinical equipoise is almost universally viewed as deriving its moral force from norms that are internal to the doctor–patient relationship. In particular, the equipoise requirement is traditionally supported as a means of reconciling the demands of sound scientific practice with the physician's therapeutic obligation. The moral force of the practical test outlined here, however, is grounded in a different source, namely, in the claim that it represents a requirement that is necessary to justify the conduct of scientific research as one element of a larger social division of labor that must be justifiable to each of the individual members of the community whose interests that division of labor is intended to serve.

Similarly, the equipoise requirement is sometimes applied to entire trial populations, whereas the above practical test is to be applied to each prospective trial participant individually. The reason for this is simply that conflict or uncertainty about the relative therapeutic merits of a set of interventions may exist for some individuals and not for others, depending on their particular clinical characteristics.

The above test is also explicit in distinguishing between uncertainty that arises from a state of agnosticism and uncertainty that arises from a state of conflict. Briefly, clinical agnosticism refers to the situation in which the expert medical community as a whole is in agreement that there are not sufficient grounds to make a definitive judgment as to the relative therapeutic merits of a set of interventions for a particular patient. Such a situation might arise, for example, in the case of a new, investigational intervention for a condition that is currently untreatable. Clinical conflict exists, however, when expert clinicians have definite opinions about the superiority of one intervention over another, for example, but their opinions are in conflict, with one physician (or set of physicians) preferring intervention A over B for patient P and another preferring B over A for P. According to the standard elaborated above, it would be permissible to offer to P the option of participating in a clinical trial in which she would be randomized to either A or B because both interventions are regarded as admissible in this scenario.

Although this very brief sketch requires significant additional elaboration, it is nonetheless sufficient to discriminate between the cases of sham surgery that were described above. In particular, it highlights as salient two significant differences between case 1, on the one hand, and cases 2 and 3 on the other.

First, arthroscopic surgery for osteoarthritis of the knee is the subject of genuine conflict in the clinical community, with a significant portion of practitioners offering this intervention to their patients and a significant portion of the expert medical community either uncertain about or affirmatively skeptical of the therapeutic merits of this intervention. In such a case, it may be permissible to perform what is referred to as an "explanatory" trial that is capable of passing the practical test articulated above.[7] In such trials, the goal is to identify which specific components of a procedure are responsible for its causal efficacy. Such a trial might pass the above test if a reasonable minority of reputable medical experts perceive some therapeutic merits to the actual arthroscopic procedure but disagree about whether these benefits result from actual débridement and lavage or from the "experience of surgery." If this were the case, then this particular sham-surgery control might be admissible on the grounds that some experts believe that it offers the prospect of a benefit that would not be received in a no-treatment arm with fewer risks than those that are associated with the actual procedure. Randomization to this arm would not provide subjects with a level of care or protection for their basic interests that falls below what is shown for subjects who seek care directly.[8]

Such a justification does not seem to be available in cases 2 and 3. In these cases, the operative clinical question is whether the new interventions being proposed provide a net therapeutic advantage over the unaugmented existing standard of care. Before it would be permissible to answer the explanatory question of which elements of these interventions are responsible for their causal efficacy, therefore, it must first be established that these interventions are efficacious in a way that makes them attractive as clinical interventions.

Second, there is an alternative prima facie case for the permissibility of the sham-surgery control in case 1. This approach has several components: (1) The state of conflict in the clinical community in case 1 makes both the procedure and no-treatment admissible interventions. (2) The operational criterion and the practical test articulated above each relate to the basic interests of trial participants and not to their broader set of personal interests; in this case, the risks associated with the sham-surgery control are largely limited to harms that pose the most credible or material threat to the personal and not the basic interests of trial participants. (3) Finally, the risks to the personal interests of subjects that are posed by the sham-surgery control in this case have been minimized as far as is consistent with preserving the blind of the study. Together, these considerations support the prima facie claim that it would be permissible to offer a trial with this risk profile to subjects on the grounds that it provides equal regard for their basic interests and for the basic interests of other community members while allowing participants to decide whether the risks that the trial poses to their personal interests are acceptable in light of its scientific goals.

This alternative prima facie case is more difficult to make in support of case 3. In particular, it is difficult to see the risks associated with this sham surgery as limited to the personal interests of participants. In part, this is due to the much higher ratio of surgery to sham in this control. That is to say, unlike case 1 where the sham surgery involved much more sham or theater, the sham surgery in this case is actually very invasive; holes are drilled through the skull, a catheter attached to an access port is inserted into the subject's head, and at regular intervals for six months saline injections are delivered to the subject's brain. In large part, however, this is due to the fact that the anticipated adverse effects associated with this control constitute more significant impediments to the functionality of subjects whose abilities to pursue their particular life projects is already being restricted by a degenerative illness.

It may be the case, however, that this sort of alternate prima case could be used to support something similar to the trial that was conducted in case 2. To build such a case, one would have to show that the risks associated with the sham surgery have been limited to harms that pose the most credible or material threat to the personal interests of subjects and that the remaining risks to the personal interests of participants had been reduced as far as possible, consistent with effectuating a blinded study. This might be done not only by utilizing partial burr holes that do not go completely through the skull but also by substituting placebo substances for any of the antibiotics or other medications whose provision cannot be justified by their therapeutic merits for the recipient. Generally speaking, the clearer it becomes that the risks associated with the sham-surgery control are limited to the personal interests of participants and that they have been reduced as far as is consistent with the integrity of the trial design, the greater the prima facie case that can

be made in support of the trial. In such cases, offering the option of participating in such a trial is consistent with a regard for the basic interests of participants that is equal to that which is being shown for the interests of future
beneficiaries that motivates the research in the first place.

As it actually stands, however, the trial in case 2 does not meet the conditions necessary for justification under either of the approaches sketched
above. Clearly, the framework that has been articulated here requires both
further refinement and clarification as well as a more substantial philosophical defense. In particular, significantly greater attention will have to be paid
to the distinction between basic and personal interests. Nevertheless, even
this relatively rudimentary sketch is sufficient to highlight some of the features of sham-surgery controls that can make them morally problematic. In
particular, the affirmative risks that are associated with sham surgeries can
endanger the basic interests of trial participants in a way that is not consistent with the same kind of respect and regard that motivates the very quest
to advance the boundaries of scientific understanding for the benefit of future persons.

## NOTES

1. For example, compare Freedman 1990 and Rothman and Michels 1994 with Miller and
Brody 2002.
2. 56 Federal Register 28012, 45 CFR 46.
3. For a general elaboration of this criticism against Miller's proposed standard and a defense of equipoise against some of his recent criticisms, see London 2006.
4. For a defense of this claim, see Rawls 1982.
5. For further discussion, see London 2003, 2006.
6. For a fuller elaboration of the differences between the view articulated here and Freedman's position, and for a general defense of this particular understanding of equipoise, see London 2006a.
7. On the difference between pragmatic and explanatory trials, see Schwartz, Flamant, and
Lellouch 1980. On the relevance of this distinction to the evaluation of trials involving a sham
surgery control, see London and Kadane 2002.
8. This argument is elaborated more fully in London and Kadane 2003. There, we emphasize
that although an argument of this form may be sufficient to justify the conduct of this trial, we
remain skeptical about whether the disagreement in the medical community over the therapeutic merits of this trial was actually grounded in an assessment of the available data.

## REFERENCES

Bower, Vicki. 2003. The ethics of innovation: Should innovative surgery be exempt from clinical
    trials and regulations? *EMBO Reports* 4 (4): 338–40.
Clark, Peter A. 2002. Placebo surgery for Parkinson's disease: Do the benefits outweigh the
    risks? *Journal of Law, Medicine & Ethics* 30 (1): 58–68.
Dekkers, Wim, and Gerard Boer. 2001. Sham neurosurgery in patients with Parkinson's disease:
    Is it morally acceptable? *Journal of Medical Ethics* 27: 151–56.

Freedman, Benjamin. 1987. Equipoise and the ethics of clinical research. *New England Journal of Medicine* 317: 141–45.

———. 1990. Placebo-controlled trials and the logic of clinical purpose. *IRB* 12 (6): 1–6.

Freeman, Thomas B., Dorothy E. Vawter, Paul E. Leaverton, James H. Godbold, Robert A. Hauser, Christopher G. Goetz, and C. Warren Olanow. 1999. Use of placebo surgery in controlled trials of a cellular-based therapy for Parkinson's disease. *New England Journal of Medicine* 341 (13): 988–92.

Horng, Sam, and Franklin G. Miller. 2002. Is placebo surgery unethical? *New England Journal of Medicine* 347 (2): 137–39.

Jonas, Hans. 1969. Philosophical reflections on experimenting with human subjects. *Daedalus* 98 (2): 219–47.

Kim, Scott Y. H. 2003. The sham surgery debate and the moral complexity of risk-benefit analysis. *American Journal of Bioethics* 3 (4): 68–70.

London, Alex John. 2003. Threats to the common good: Biochemical weapons and human subjects research. *Hastings Center Report* 33 (5): 17–25.

———. 2005. Does research ethics rest on a mistake? The common good, reasonable risk and social justice. *American Journal of Bioethics* 5 (1): 37–39.

———. 2006. Clinical equipoise: Foundational requirement or fundamental error. In *Oxford Handbook of Bioethics*, ed. Bonnie Steinbock. New York: Oxford University Press.

London, Alex John, and Joseph B. Kadane. 2002. Placebos that harm: Sham surgery controls in clinical trials. *Statistical Methods in Medical Research* 11 (5): 413–27.

———. 2003. Sham surgery and genuine standards of care: Can the two be reconciled? *American Journal of Bioethics* 3 (4): 61–64.

Macklin, Ruth. 1999. The ethical problems with sham surgery in clinical research. *New England Journal of Medicine* 341 (13): 992–96.

Miller, Franklin G. 2003. Sham surgery: An ethical analysis. *American Journal of Bioethics* 3 (4): 41–48.

Miller, Franklin G., and Howard Brody. 2002. What makes placebo-controlled trials unethical? *American Journal of Bioethics* 2 (2): 3–9.

Moseley, J. Bruce, Kimberly O'Malley, Nancy J. Petersen, Terri J. Menke, Baruch A. Brody, David H. Kuykendall, John C. Hollingsworth, Carol M. Ashton, and Nelda P. Wray. 2002. A controlled trial of arthroscopic surgery for osteoarthritis of the knee. *New England Journal of Medicine* 347 (2): 81–88.

Nutt, J. G., K. J. Burchiel, C. L. Comella, J. Jankovic, A. E. Lang, E. R. Laws Jr., A. M. Lozano, R. D. Penn, R. K. Simpson Jr., M. Stacy, and G. F. Wooten. 2003. Randomized, double-blind trial of glial cell line-derived neurotrophic factor (GDNF) in PD. *Neurology* 60: 69–73.

Rawls, John. 1982. Social unity and primary goods. In *Utilitarianism and beyond*, ed. Amartya Sen and Bernard Williams, 159–85. Cambridge: Cambridge University Press.

Reitsma, Angelique M., and Jonathan D. Moreno. 2002. Ethical regulations for innovative surgery: The last frontier? *Journal of the American College of Surgeons* 194 (6): 792–801.

Rothman, Kenneth J., and Karen B. Michels. 1994. The continuing unethical use of placebo controls. *New England Journal of Medicine* 331: 394–98.

Schwartz, D., R. Flamant, and J. Lellouch. 1980. *Clinical trials*, trans. M. J. R. Healy. London: Academic Press.

Weijer, Charles. 2000. The ethical analysis of risk. *Journal of Law, Medicine & Ethics* 28: 344–61.

———. 2002. I need a placebo like I need a hole in the head. *Journal of Law, Medicine & Ethics* 30 (1): 69–72.

# Suggestions
# for Further Reading

## MALE CIRCUMCISION AND FEMALE GENITAL CUTTING

Benatar, David, and Michael Benatar. "How Not to Argue about Circumcision." *American Journal of Bioethics* 3, no. 2 (Spring 2003): W1–W9. Available at http://www.bioethics.net/journal/pdf/3_2_LT_w01_Benetar.pdf.

Gollaher, David L. *Circumcision: A History of the World's Most Controversial Surgery.* New York: Basic Books, 2000.

Kopelman, Loretta. "Female Circumcision and Genital Mutilation." In *Encyclopedia of Applied Ethics*, ed. Ruth Chadwick, 2: 249–59. San Diego: Academic Press, 1998.

Shell-Duncan, Bettina, and Ylva Hernlund, eds. *Female "Circumcision" in Africa: Culture, Controversy and Change.* Boulder, CO: Lynne Rienner, 2000.

Somerville, Margaret. "Altering Baby Boys' Bodies: The Ethics of Infant Male Circumcision." In *The Ethical Canary: Science, Society, and the Human Spirit*, 202–19. Toronto: Viking, 2000.

Szasz, Thomas. "Routine Neonatal Circumcision: Symbol of the Birth of the Therapeutic State." *Journal of Medicine and Philosophy* 21 (1996): 137–48.

## SEX ASSIGNMENT AND SEX REASSIGNMENT SURGERY

Chase, Cheryl. "Surgical Progress Is Not the Answer to Intersexuality." *Journal of Clinical Ethics* 9, no. 4 (Winter 1998): 385–92.

Colapinto, John. *As Nature Made Him: The Boy Who Was Raised as a Girl.* New York: Harper-Collins, 2000.

Diamond, Milton, and Keith Sigmundson. "Management of Intersexuality: Guidelines for Dealing with Persons with Ambiguous Genitalia." *Archives of Pediatrics and Adolescent Medicine* 151 (October 1997): 1046–50.

Draper, Heather. "Transsexuals and Werewolves: The Ethical Acceptability of the Sex-Change Operation." In *Ethics, Technology and Medicine*, ed. David Braine and Harry Lesser, 114–22. Avebury, England: Aldershot, 1988.

Dreger, Alice Domurat. *Hermaphrodites and the Medical Invention of Sex*. Cambridge, MA: Harvard University Press, 1998.

Elliott, Carl. "Why Can't We Go On as Three?" *Hastings Center Report* 28, no. 3 (May–June 1998): 36–39.

Goveman, Sherri A. "The Hanukkah Bush: Ethical Implications in the Clinical Management of Intersex." *Journal of Clinical Ethics* 9, no. 4 (Winter 1998): 356–59.

Kipnis, Kenneth, and Milton Diamond. "Pediatric Ethics and the Surgical Assignment of Sex." *Journal of Clinical Ethics* 9, no. 4 (Winter 1998): 398–410.

Schober, Justine Marut. "A Surgeon's Response to the Intersex Controversy." *Journal of Clinical Ethics* 9, no. 4 (Winter 1998): 393–97.

Minto, Catherine, L. M. Liao, C. R. Woodhouse, P. G. Ransley, and S. M. Creighton. "The Effect of Clitoral Surgery on Sexual Outcome in Individuals Who Have Intersex Conditions with Ambiguous Genitalia: A Cross-Sectional Study." *Lancet* 361, no. 9365 (April 12, 2003): 1252–57.

Wilson, Bruce E., and William G. Reiner. "Management of Intersex: A Shifting Paradigm." *Journal of Clinical Ethics* 9, no. 4 (Winter 1998): 360–69.

## SEPARATING CONJOINED TWINS

Cywes, S., A. J. W. Millar, H. Rode, and R. A. Brown. "Conjoined Twins: The Cape Town Experience." *Pediatric Surgery International* 12, no. 4 (April 1997): 234–48.

Dreger, Alice Domurat. *One of Us: Conjoined Twins and the Future of Normal*. Cambridge, MA: Harvard University Press, 2004.

Sheldon, Sally, and Stephen Wilkinson. "Conjoined Twins: The Legality and Ethics of Sacrifice." *Medical Law Review* 5 (Summer 1997): 149–71.

Thomasma, David, J. Muraskas, P. Marshall, T. Myers, P. Tomich, and J. O'Neill. "The Ethics of Caring for Conjoined Twins: The Lakeberg Twins." *Hastings Center Report* 26, no. 4 (July–August 1996): 4–12.

## LIMB AND FACE TRANSPLANTATION

Benatar, David, and Don Hudson. "A Tale of Two Novel Transplants Not Done: The Ethics of Limb Allografts." *British Medical Journal* 324 (April 20, 2002): 971–73.

Dubernard, Jean-Michel, E. Owen, G. Herzberg, M. Lanzetta, X. Martin, H. Kapila, M. Dawahra, and N. S. Hakim. "Human Hand Allograft: Report on First Six Months." *Lancet* 353, no. 9161 (April 17, 1999): 1315–20.

Jones, Jon W., Scott A. Gruber, John H. Barker, and Warren C. Breidenbach. "Successful Hand Transplantation—One-Year Follow-Up." *New England Journal of Medicine* 343, no. 7 (August 17, 2000): 468–73.

Klapheke, Martin M., Carrie Marcell, Greg Taliaferro, and Beth Creamer. "Psychiatric Assessment of Candidates for Hand Transplantation." *Microsurgery* 20, no. 8 (2000): 453–57.

Simmons, Paul D. "Ethical Considerations in Composite Tissue Allotransplantation." *Microsurgery* 20, no. 8 (2000): 458–65.

## COSMETIC SURGERY

Davis, Kathy. *Dubious Equalities and Embodied Differences*. Lanham, MD: Rowman & Littlefield, 2003.

————. *Reshaping the Female Body: The Dilemmas of Cosmetic Surgery.* New York: Routledge, 1995.

Gilman, Sander L. *Making the Body Beautiful: A Cultural History of Aesthetic Surgery.* Princeton, NJ: Princeton University Press, 1999.

Hyman, David. "Aesthetics and Ethics: The Implications of Cosmetic Surgery." *Perspectives in Biology and Medicine* 33, no. 2 (Winter 1990): 190–202.

Kirkland, Anna, and Rosemarie Tong. "Working within Contradiction: The Possibility of Feminist Cosmetic Surgery." *Journal of Clinical Ethics* 7, no. 2 (Summer 1996): 151–59.

Miller, Franklin G., Howard Brody, and Kevin C. Chung. "Cosmetic Surgery and the Internal Morality of Medicine." *Cambridge Quarterly of Healthcare Ethics* 9 (2000): 353–64.

## PLACEBO SURGERY

Clark, Chalmers C. "The Physician's Role, 'Sham Surgery', and Trust: A Conflict of Duties." *American Journal of Bioethics* 3, no. 4 (Fall 2003): 57–58.

Clark, Peter A. "Sham Surgery: To Cut or Not to Cut—That Is the Ethical Dilemma." *American Journal of Bioethics* 3, no. 4 (Fall 2003): 66–68.

Freeman, Thomas B., Dorothy E. Vawter, Paul E. Leaverton, James H. Godbold, Robert A. Hauser, Christopher G. Goetz, and C. Warren Olanow. "Use of Placebo Surgery in Controlled Trials of a Cellular-Based Therapy for Parkinson's Disease." *New England Journal of Medicine* 341, no. 13 (September 23, 1999): 988–92.

Kim, Scott Y. H. "The Sham Surgery Debate and the Moral Complexity of Risk-Benefit Analysis." *American Journal of Bioethics* 3, no. 4 (Fall 2003): 68–70.

London, Alex John, and Joseph B. Kadane. "Placebos That Harm: Sham Surgery Controls in Clinical Trials." *Statistical Methods in Medical Research* 11 (2002): 413–27.

————. "Sham Surgery and Genuine Standards of Care: Can the Two be Reconciled?" *American Journal of Bioethics* 3, no. 4 (Fall 2003): 61–64.

Macklin, Ruth. "The Ethical Problems with Sham Surgery in Clinical Research." *New England Journal of Medicine* 341, no. 13 (September 23, 1999): 992–96.

Miller, Franklin G. "Sham Surgery: An Ethical Analysis." *American Journal of Bioethics* 3, no. 4 (Fall 2003): 41–48.

Rhodes, Rosamond. "An Innovative Paradigm for Clinical Research." *American Journal of Bioethics* 3, no. 4 (Fall 2003): 59–61.

# Index

*Page references listed in italics refer to textboxes on that page.*

# About the
# Editor and Contributors

**Françoise Baylis**, Canada Research Chair in Bioethics and Philosophy, is professor of medicine and philosophy at Dalhousie University, Halifax, Nova Scotia, Canada.

**David Benatar** is associate professor of philosophy at the University of Cape Town, South Africa.

**Michael Benatar** is assistant professor of neurology at Emory University, Atlanta, Georgia, United States.

**Leslie Cannold** is senior research fellow at the Centre for Applied Philosophy and Public Ethics at the University of Melbourne, Australia.

**Stephen Coleman** is research fellow at the Centre for Applied Philosophy and Public Ethics, Charles Sturt University, Canberra ACT, Australia.

**Dena S. Davis** is professor of law at Cleveland-Marshall College of Law, Cleveland State University, Ohio, United States.

**Donna Dickenson** is professor of medical ethics and humanities and executive director of the Birkbeck Institute for the Humanities at the University of London, England.

**Heather Draper** is senior lecturer at the Centre for Biomedical Ethics at the University of Birmingham, England.

**Neil Evans** is a doctoral student at the Centre for Biomedical Ethics at the University of Birmingham, England.

**Richard Hull** is lecturer in philosophy at the National University of Ireland, Galway, Ireland.

**Hilde Lindemann** is associate professor of philosophy at Michigan State University, East Lansing, Michigan, United States.

**Alex John London** is associate professor of philosophy at Carnegie Mellon University, Pittsburgh, Pennsylvania, United States.

**David Neil** is lecturer in philosophy at the University of Wollongong, Wollongong, New South Wales, Australia.

**Julian Savulescu** is Uehiro Chair in Practical Ethics at the University of Oxford, Oxford, England.

**Merle Spriggs** is ethicist and postdoctoral researcher at Murdoch Children's Research Institute, and honorary fellow at the Centre for the Study of Health and Society, at the University of Melbourne, Australia.

**Rosemarie Tong** is distinguished professor in healthcare ethics at the University of North Carolina, Charlotte, North Carolina, United States.

**David Wasserman** is research scholar at the Institute for Philosophy and Public Policy at the University of Maryland, College Park, Maryland, United States.

**Guy Widdershoven** is professor of ethics of health care at the University of Maastricht, Maastricht, the Netherlands.

**Stephen Wilkinson** is senior lecturer at the Centre for Professional Ethics at Keele University, Keele, Staffordshire, England.